Sports, Health and Exercise Medicine

Edited by Samuel Honório, Marco Batista, João Serrano and Maria-Raquel G. Silva

Published in London, United Kingdom

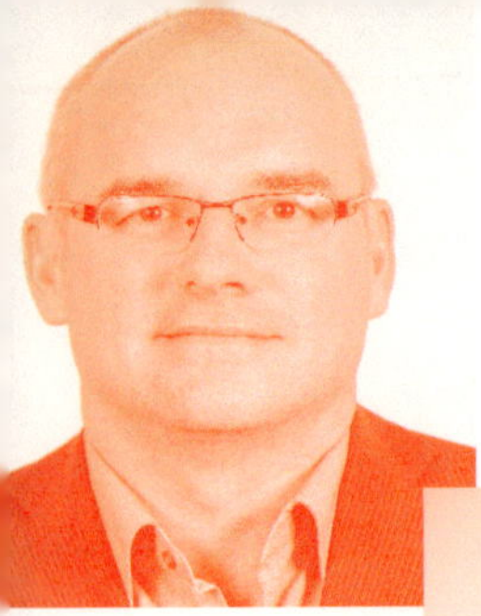
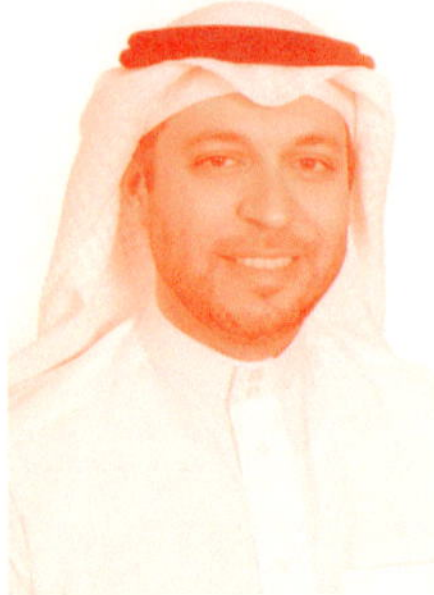
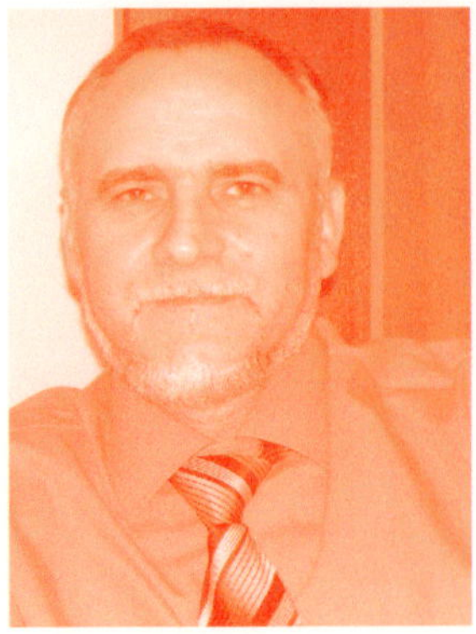
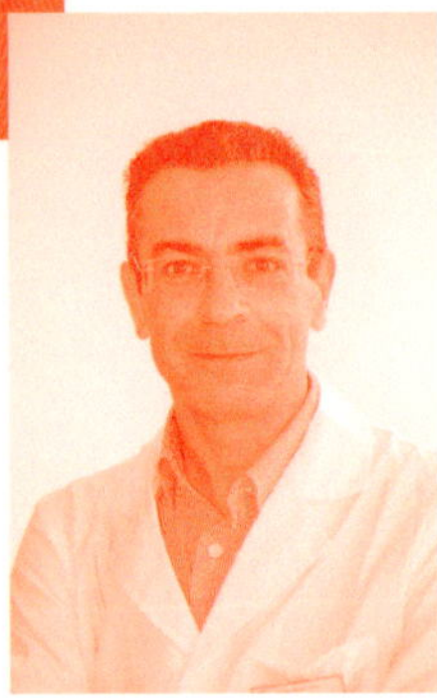
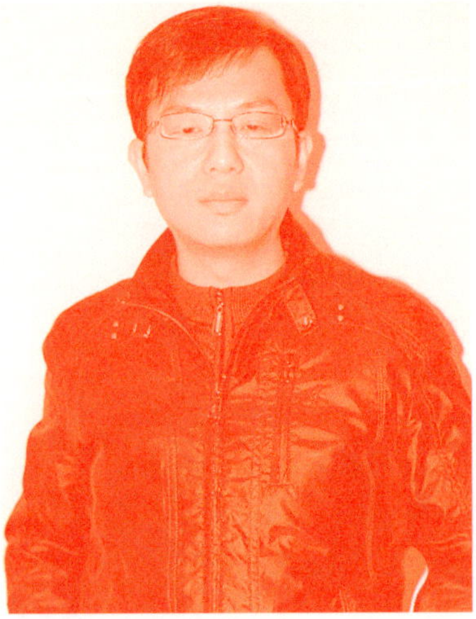
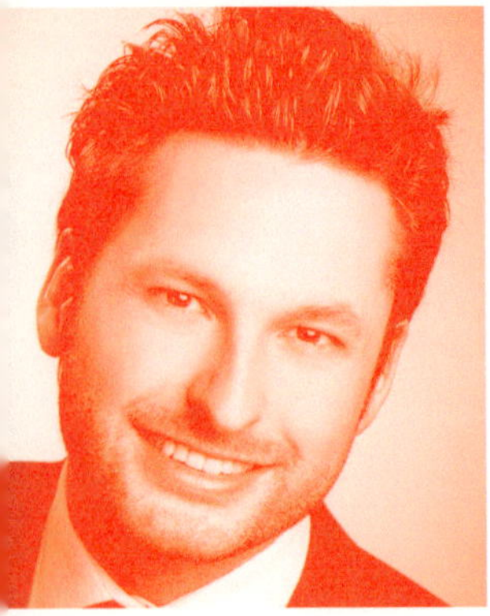
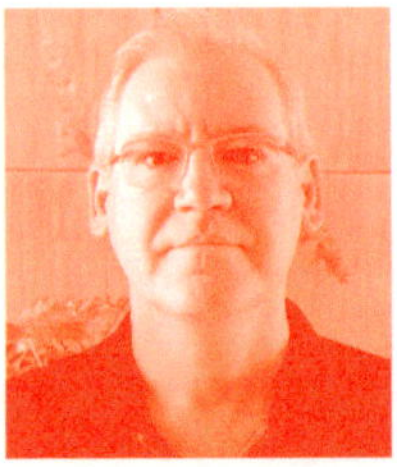

IntechOpen

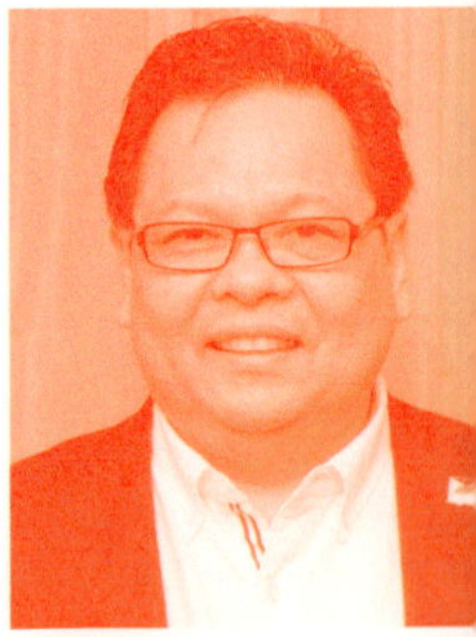
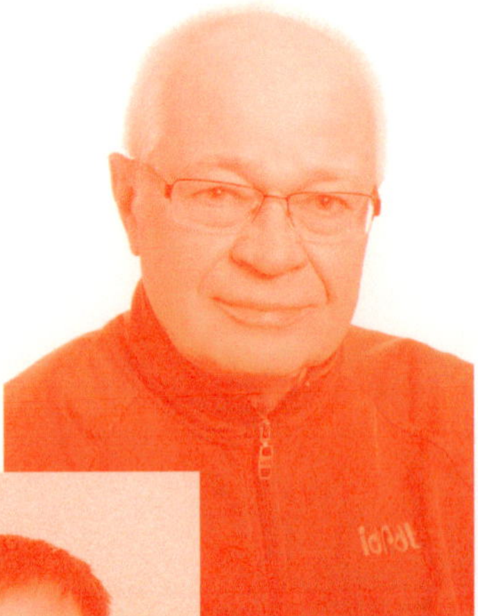
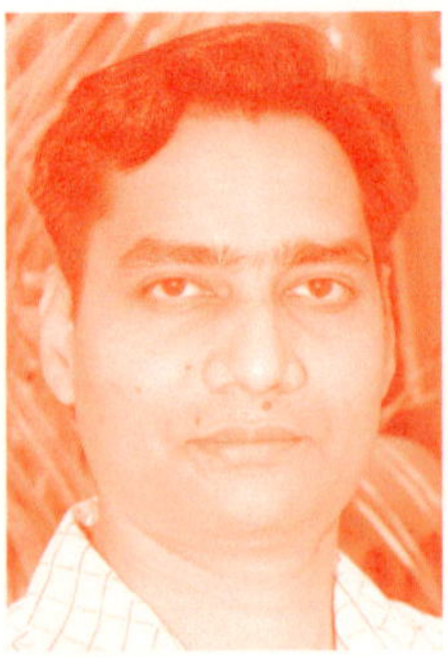
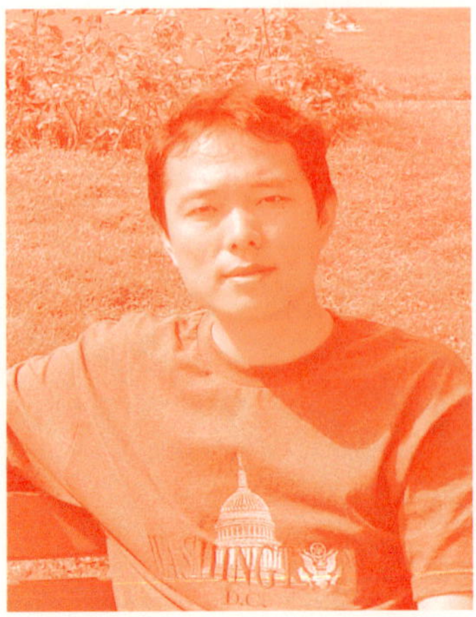
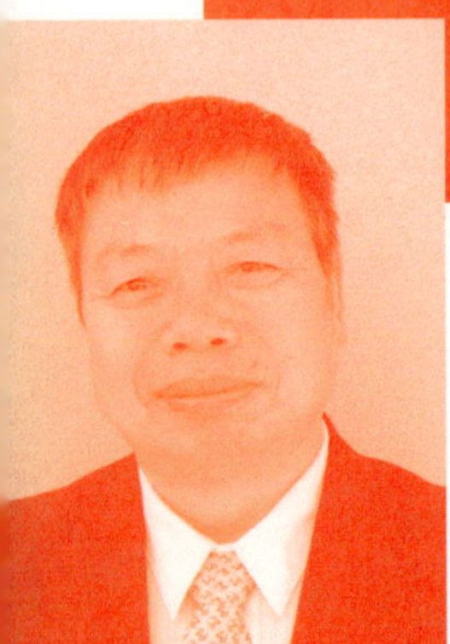
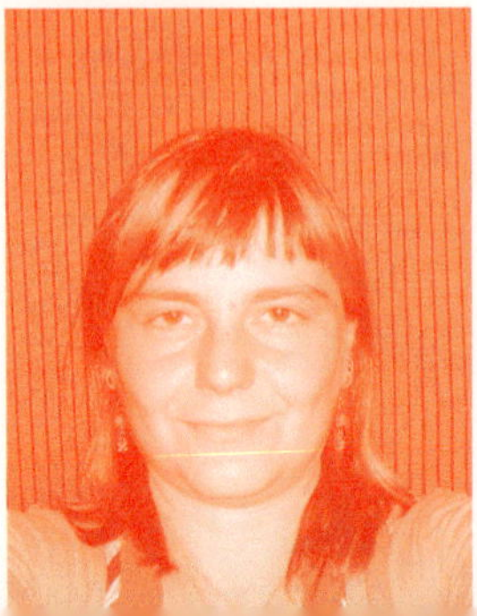

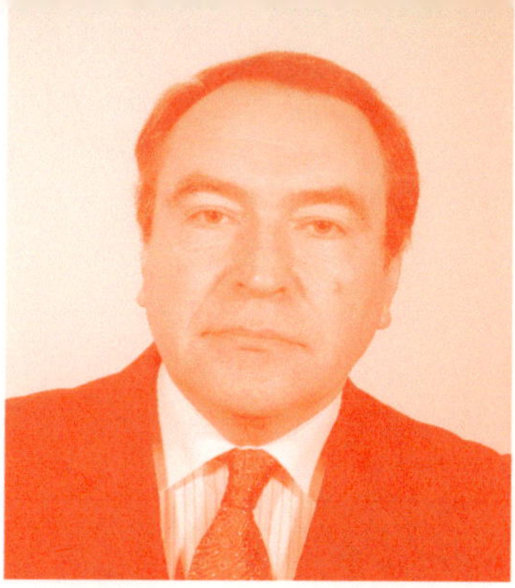
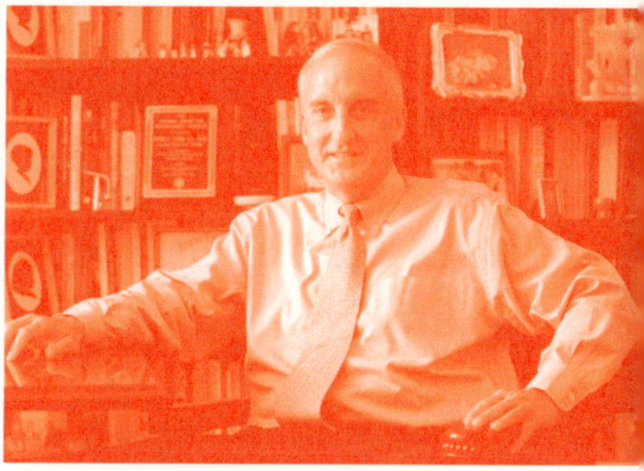
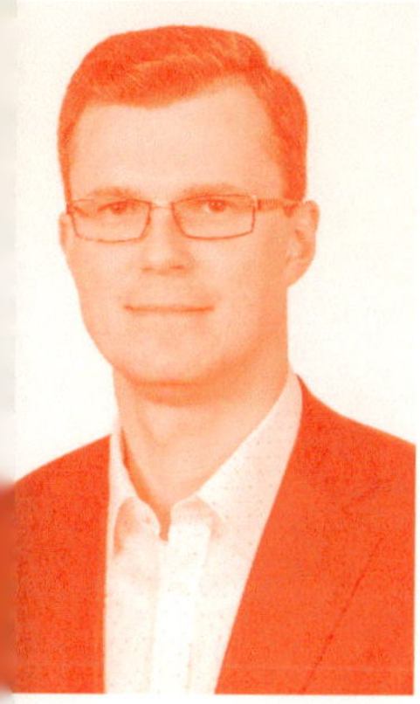
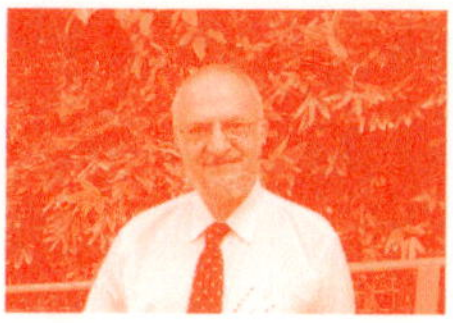
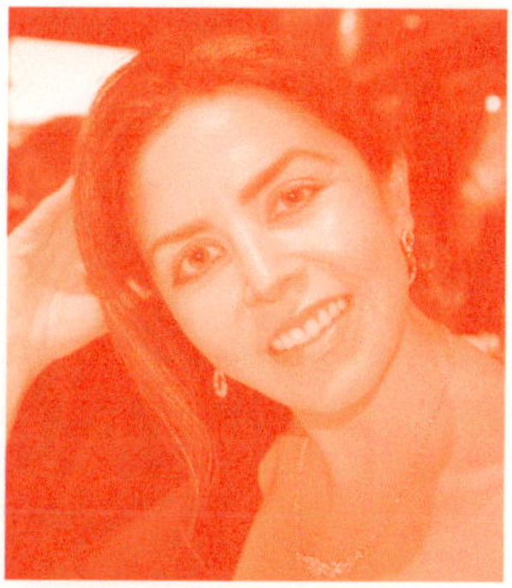

Supporting open minds since 2005

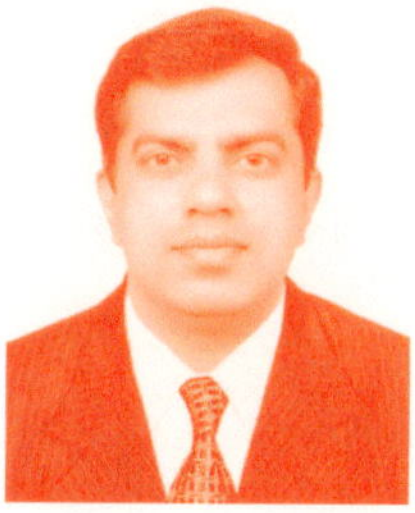
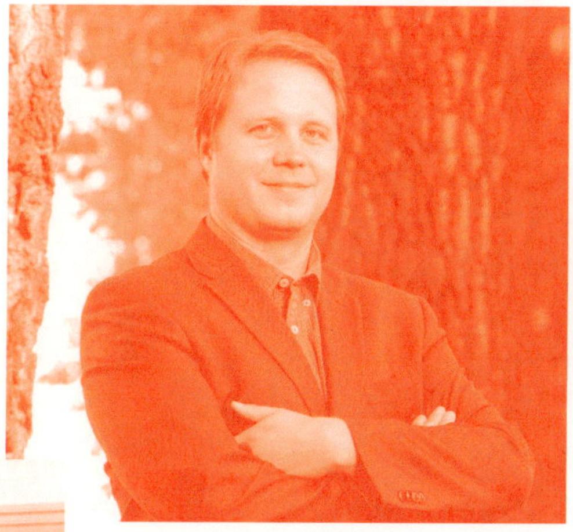
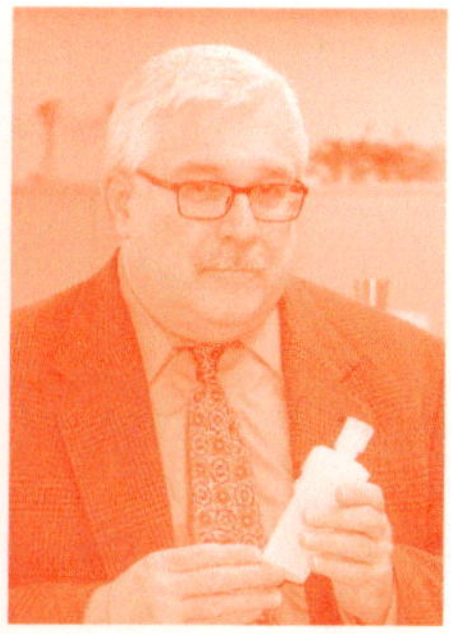
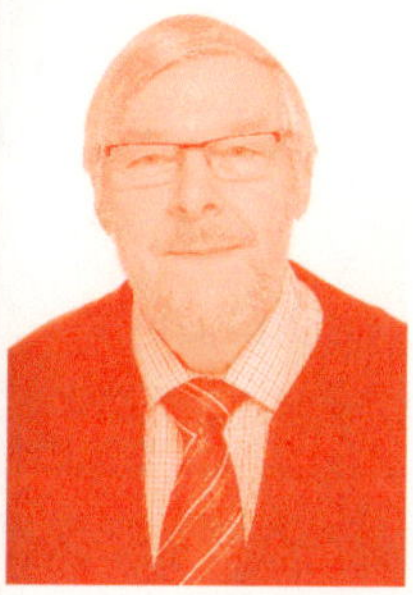
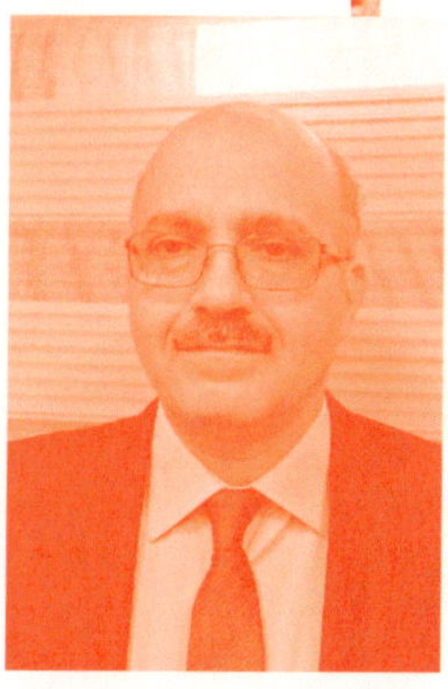
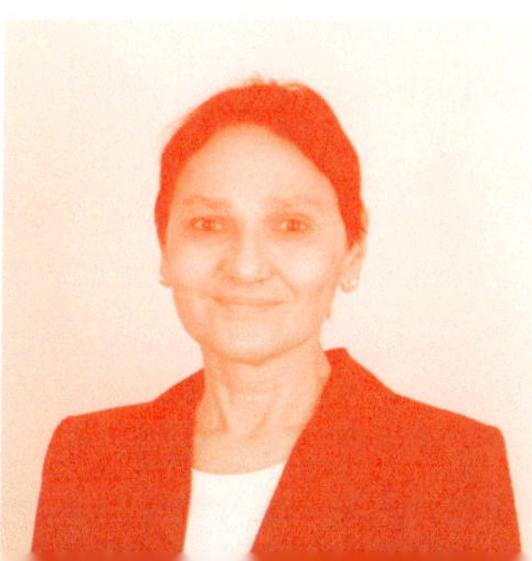
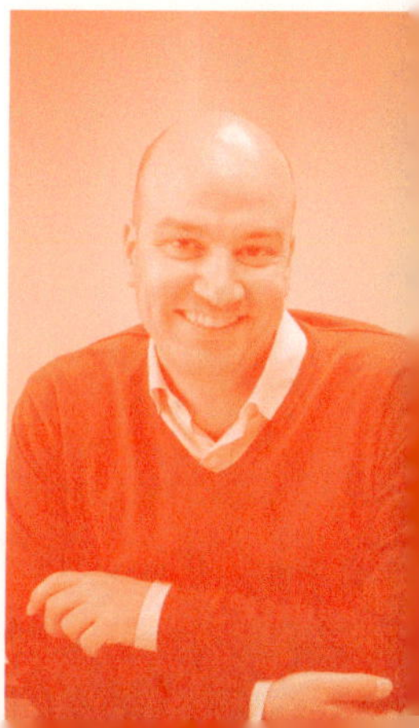

Sports, Health and Exercise Medicine
http://dx.doi.org/10.5772/intechopen.83149
Edited by Samuel Honório, Marco Batista, João Serrano and Maria-Raquel G. Silva

Contributors
Victor Moskvin, Danielle Leong, Felipe Hardt, Rafael Cristiano Geiss Santos, Olga Lakomy, Aleksandra Zebrowska, Robert Trybulski, Artur Gołaś, Jeeser Almeida, Keemilyn Silva, Suzilene Ormond, Dayanne Sarah Lima-Borges, Murilo Nogueira, Konstantin Popenko, Nina Moskvina, Vladimir Nurgaleev, Zhanna Lukyanchikova, Vladimir Nepopalov, Elena Romanina, Vladimir Sopov

First published in London, United Kingdom, 2020 by IntechOpen
IntechOpen is the global imprint of INTECHOPEN LIMITED, registered in England and Wales, registration number: 11086078, 7th floor, 10 Lower Thames Street, London, EC3R 6AF, United Kingdom
Printed in Croatia

British Library Cataloguing-in-Publication Data
A catalogue record for this book is available from the British Library

Additional hard and PDF copies can be obtained from orders@intechopen.com

Sports, Health and Exercise Medicine
Edited by Samuel Honório, Marco Batista, João Serrano and Maria-Raquel G. Silva
p. cm.
Print ISBN 978-1-83880-399-5
Online ISBN 978-1-83880-400-8
eBook (PDF) ISBN 978-1-83968-182-0

For EU product safety concerns:
IN TECH d.o.o., Prolaz Marije Krucifikse Kozulić 3, 51000 Rijeka, Croatia, info@intechopen.com or visit our website at intechopen.com.

Meet the editors

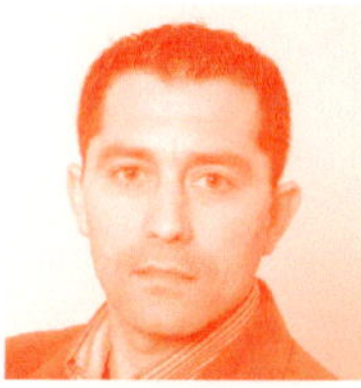

Dr. Samuel Honório is a full-time teacher in the Polytechnic Institute of Castelo Branco – Higher School of Education, Portugal. He is a member of the Sports and Well Being Department and in SHERU (Sport, Health and Exercise Research Unit). He serves as an Adjunct Professor, has a PhD in Sport Sciences and a Post-doctorate graduation in Physical Activity and Health, with a specialty in exercise and health. He also has a Masters degree in Education Sciences and a Bachelor's degree in teaching physical activity. He is also an author and co-author of several books and articles in the field.

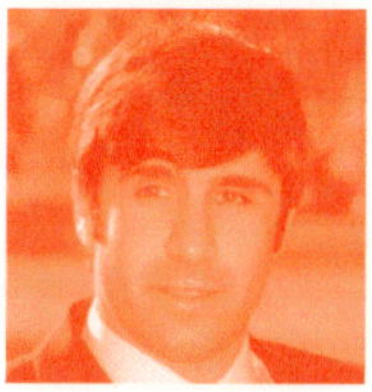

Dr. Marco Batista is a fulltime teacher at the Polytechnic Institute of Castelo Branco - Higher School of Education, Portugal. He is a member of the Sports and Well Being Department and SHERU (Sport, Health and Exercise Research Unit). He has obtained his PhD in Educational Sciences from the University of Extremadura (Spain). He is now a teacher at the Polytechnic Institute of Castelo Branco, being the teacher of the curricular unit in the Bachelor Degree of Sports and Physical Activity and in the Master Degree of Physical Activity. He has served as a supervisor of several master theses on Sport Sciences, and an author and co-author of articles in indexed peer-reviewed journals.

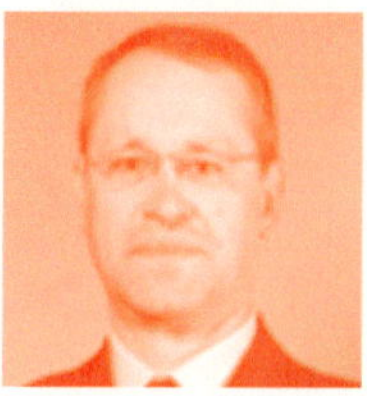

João Júlio de Matos Serrano has a PhD in Human Motricity from the Faculty of Human Kinetics at the Technical University of Lisbon. He has been a teacher in the scientific area of sport and well-being at the Higher School of Education of the Polytechnic Institute of Castelo Branco since 1991. He is the Director of the Higher School of Education and Integrated Researcher and Co -coordinator of the Sport, Health & Exercise Research Unit (SHERU), Research Unit of the Polytechnic Institute of Castelo Branco. He is an author and editor of 10 books and 45 book chapters, and has published scientific articles in international journals with peer review. He has participated as a lecturer in many national and international congresses, was a member of the scientific committee of more than 30 congresses/seminars, coordinated several projects, and has participated in the organization of many scientific events.

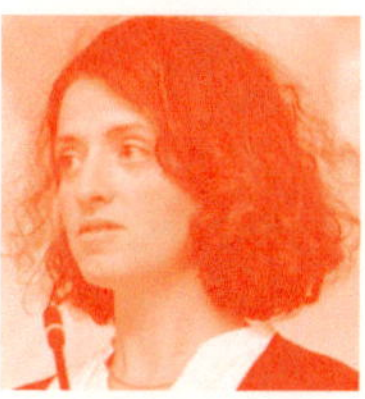

Maria-Raquel G. Silva is an Associate Professor of Nutrition and Dietetics at the Faculty of Health Sciences-University Fernando Pessoa in Porto. She is a Senior Researcher in the Research Centre for Anthropology and Health-Human Biology, Health and Society Group-University of Coimbra and in the Comprehensive Health Research Centre-Group of Sleep, Chronobiology and Sleep Disorders-Nova Medical School, University of Lisbon. She is an expert in nutrition for the Scientific Committee of the Gymnastics Federation of Portugal as well as being an ex-rhythmic gymnast, coach and international judge. She achieved her Pos-Doc in Neurosciences (Institute of Molecular Medicine-Medical Faculty of Lisbon), Ph.D. in Nutrition Sciences and has a Licentiate Degree in Sport and Physical Education (University of Porto). Her research areas are nutrition and metabolic diseases, neurosciences and physical exercise.

Contents

Preface

Sport is made by people and is for people, as it is a multidisciplinary process involving athletes, coaches, clinical staff, families, managers, and other institutional supporters, such as academia and industry.

We have been working in sport for almost 40 years and the opportunity to be in daily contact with athletes and coaches has given us the will to study them harder in order to promote the athlete's health and performance and to ensure the best training regimes.

Fortunately, the increasing number of scientific disciplines surrounding sport, namely sports medicine, physiology, neurophysiology, psychology, sports health, nutrition, biomechanics (among others) are driving sport and athletes into safer and later sport experiences, which is in fact the added value of this book.

This book presents a diversity of themes related to sports medicine and health varying from clinical issues, such as sports injuries to specific neuropsychological aspects of the athletes' behaviour regulation and parathletes' motivation for sport practice.

The book is structured in six chapters, which combine research and clinical/exercise applications that we would like to highlight. Chapter 1 involves the study of the volitional (arbitrary) regulation of behaviour and its connections with the individual features of interhemispheric asymmetries in sports activities practice. Chapter 2 addresses the role of one important professional in sport, which is the Sport and Exercise Medicine physician, and his specific training, skills, and abilities from recreational sports to elite level and as a healthy lifestyle promoter. Chapter 3 discusses the pathophysiology of a mild traumatic brain injury or sport-related concussion sustained during sports participation and presents the scientific evidence-based acute screening and detection methods available and general guidelines for recovery and active rehabilitation. Chapter 4 is focused on the pathophysiology of the knee-dislocation and strategies to increase strength and endurance training in rehabilitation. Chapter 5 is practice-oriented to the adaptive responses inherent to exercise training on cardiac remodelling. Chapter 6 reports results on the motivation of Russian highly qualified parathletes from three different regions.

This comprehensive volume is very appealing, which will be also recognised by sports and health professionals, who need further support in their daily work with athletes and coaches, in particular. It is also attractive to researchers and students interested in sport and health related areas.

Samuel Honório, Marco Batista and João Serrano
SHERU - Sports, Health and Exercise Research Unit,
Polytechnic Institute of Castelo Branco,
Portugal

Maria-Raquel G. Silva,
Faculty of Health Sciences,
University Fernando Pessoa,
Porto, Portugal

Research Centre for Anthropology and Health,
Group of Human Biology, Health and Society,
University of Coimbra,
Coimbra, Portugal

Comprehensive Health Research Centre,
Group of Sleep, Chronobiology and Sleep Disorders,
Nova Medical School,
University of Lisbon,
Lisbon, Portugal

Section 1

Sport and Injuries Preventions

Chapter 1

Sports-Related Traumatic Brain Injury: Screening and Management

Danielle Leong

Abstract

Mild traumatic brain injury (mTBI) sustained during sports participation, also known as sport-related concussion, has received increasing attention due in large part to the growing public awareness of the risks of head injury exposure in sports and the long-term consequences of repetitive head trauma. This chapter will review the latest understanding of concussion pathophysiology and provide an up to date overview of the scientific evidence-based acute screening and detection methods available for laypersons and medical professionals providing frontline assessment for athletes. Lastly, a comprehensive summary of clinical management for recovery management and approaches for active rehabilitation will be covered.

Keywords: balance, clinical management, concussion detection, eye movements, head trauma, K-D test, King-Devick test, pathophysiology, saccades, screening, recovery, recovery acceleration program, rehabilitation, mTBI, traumatic brain injury

1. Introduction

An estimated 41 million American children participate in competitive sports each year [1]. Participation in competitive sports is not without risk, however, as the Center for Disease Control reports that 2.7 million children aged 19 and under visited the emergency room annually for sports related injuries from 2001 to 2009 [2]. Specifically sports concussion is becoming an increasing public health issue as prevalence is estimated at 1.6–3.8 million annually [3]. Youth sports also contribute significantly to high rates of mild traumatic brain injury with 29% of sports related concussions happening in athletes between 16 and 19 years of age, and 40% of sports sports-related concussions occurring between 2001 and 2005 being sustained by children ages 8–13 [4, 5]. Although, cycling is the leading cause of head injury in children under the age of 14 [6], the three highest concussion rates in high school sports can be attributed to football, boys' ice hockey, and girls' soccer, with estimated rates of 76.8, 54, and 33 concussions per 100,000 athletic exposures, respectively [7]. These reports are likely underestimated as not all injured individuals seek medical care and therefore an estimated 50% of concussive injuries go unreported [8].

There is lack of a concrete and consistent definition of concussion which also creates challenges in the accuracy of sports related concussion epidemiology estimations. However, we share here the most widely accepted definition of concussion most recently published by an international consensus group [9], which is defined as:

Concussion is a brain injury and is defined as a complex pathophysiological process affecting the brain, induced by biomechanical forces. Several common features that incorporate clinical, pathologic and biomechanical injury constructs that may be utilized in defining the nature of a concussive head injury include:

1. Concussion may be caused either by a direct blow to the head, face, neck or elsewhere on the body with an "impulsive' force transmitted to the head.

2. Concussion typically results in the rapid onset of short-lived impairment of neurological function that resolves spontaneously. However, in some cases, symptoms and signs may evolve over a number of minutes to hours.

3. Concussion may result in neuropathological changes, but the acute clinical symptoms largely reflect a functional disturbance rather than a structural injury and, as such, no abnormality is seen on standard structural neuroimaging studies.

4. Concussion results in a graded set of clinical symptoms that may or may not involve loss of consciousness. Resolution of the clinical and cognitive symptoms typically follows a sequential course. However, it is important to note that in some cases symptoms may be prolonged [9].

Concussions result in a myriad of symptomatology which are generally categorized into four main domains: (1) physical (i.e. headache, dizziness, visual dysfunction), (2) cognitive (i.e. difficult with concentration and memory), (3) emotional (i.e. depression, anxiety and mood lability), (4) sleep disturbance (hypersomnia and insomnia). The most commonly reported symptoms include headache, dizziness and difficulties with concentration and memory. Symptoms are likely caused by functional, metabolic and microstructural abnormalities as routine neuroimaging is typically unhelpful at demonstrating anatomical evidence of neuropathic changes [10].

Exposure to repetitive concussion or sub-concussive impacts, in which a significant traumatic brain injury may have occurred even in the absence of visible signs or symptoms, is now recognized as having possible long-term neurological consequences, including neurodegenerative disease [11–15]. Given the growing incidence and concern around sports concussion as well as the potential long-term sequelae associated with the injury, awareness of the current understanding of the pathophysiology is vital within the general field of sports medicine. Additionally, as targeted screening and management options are becoming increasingly available, knowledge of the current evidence-based tools for effective screening and subsequent management of the injury are important.

2. Concussion pathophysiology

2.1 Biomechanics of the injury

Biomechanical forces from sports impact that result in traumatic brain injury or concussion leads to functional impairment at the level of individual cells or neurons. This abnormal cellular function results in overall neurological function impairment and may lead to microstructural and subsequent macrostructural damage.

Inertial, or acceleration loading, transmitted to the brain is a primary cause of concussive injury. Both linear and rotational accelerations cause transient increases in pressure within the brain and causes shear forces [16]. The forces and pressure experienced within the brain leads to changes at a cellular level. Neuronal axons can become quickly stretched resulting in a complex cascade of ionic, metabolic and pathophysiological events.

2.2 Metabolic cascade

Changes in intracellular ion concentrations occur due to disruption of cell membranes causing an abnormal outflux of potassium causes irregular neuronal depolarization which in turn leads to increased extracellular potassium and neurotransmitter release. Glutamate, an excitatory neurotransmitter, further promotes potassium efflux and binds to N-methyl-D-aspartate receptors which additionally allows for hyperexcitability and continued unhindered depolarization of the neuron. Simultaneously, accumulation of excitatory neurotransmitters also leads to influx of calcium which promotes proteases, reactive oxygen species and mitochondrial impairment all of which contribute to cellular dysfunction, damage and death when the neuron is unable to recover cellular stability [17, 18].

Dysfunction in the regulation of neurotransmitters as well as the inciting excitotoxicity of the neuron causes significant stress on the cellular mitochondria to maintain to energy demands through ATP production. The sodium/potassium (Na^+/K^+) pumps which require ATP struggle to maintain the cellular ion homeostasis. The glycolysis process is activated in an attempt to provide this increased energy demand which leads to accumulation of lactic acid. This lactic acid breaks down the blood-brain barrier and leads to cerebral edema [17].

2.3 Neuroinflammatory response and cerebral blood flow alterations

There is also a neuroinflammatory response that occurs after brain trauma which increases microglial cells, cytokine mediators, proteases and reactive oxygen species which promotes widespread inflammation and breakdown of the blood-brain barrier. This leads to cerebral blood flow changes [17, 18]. Other cerebral blood flow changes also occur as a result of carbon dioxide that accumulates from the metabolic changes occurring. Carbon dioxide causes decreases in vasoreactivity acutely and chronically. These changes can lead to many of the acute and chronic symptoms experienced by individuals suffering from sports-related concussion and also puts them at increased risk for subsequent head injury during this recovery period [17, 18].

2.4 Chronic pathophysiology

Repetitive traumatic brain injury exposure and sub-concussive injuries, in which a substantial injury is sustain however no outward signs or symptoms are apparent, can lead to persistent neurodegenerative changes. The acute neuroinflammatory response discussed above as well as the sustained neuroinflammation that may occur can result in the development of more permanent neurocognitive deficit symptoms and neurodegenerative changes. Additionally, diffuse axonal injury that occurs from concussive impacts can result in further neurodegenerative processes and permanent changes [17, 19].

Concussion has been linked to sequelae such as post-concussion syndrome and long-term neurodegenerative disease [14]. Studies have shown a 1.5 fold increased risk of depression and a 4.5 fold increased risk of Alzheimer's-like symptoms in patients with concussion history [11]. Pathological neurodegeneration markers typically found in Alzheimer's disease has also been seen in individuals with a history of repetitive traumatic brain injury. Although no causal relationship has yet been established, recent research also suggests that repeated head trauma may be associated with the development of chronic traumatic encephalopathy (CTE), a neuropathological neurodegenerative disease defined by abnormal phosphorylated tau accumulation in a pattern distinct from other tauopathies and believed to be caused by the series of metabolic, ionic, membrane, and cytoskeletal disturbances [12, 15, 20]. Tau, a normal structural axonal protein, can become disrupted during brain trauma and accumulate in a phosphorylated form. This further destabilizes microtubules and results in impaired axonal function [12, 15, 20].

3. Acute screening and detection methods

Since detecting early signs of sports-related concussion and timely removal from play may reduce the occurrence of second concussions and continued repetitive injury, there is an essential need for understanding and implementing practical sideline tests to aid in diagnosis. Next, we discuss current acute screening and detection methods for sports-related concussion.

3.1 Standardized assessment of concussion

The Standardized Assessment of Concussion (SAC) is used as a brief cognitive assessment by measuring orientation, immediate memory, concentration and delayed recall. An orientation score out of 5 points possible is determined from five questions: (1) What month is it?, (2) What is the date?, (3) What day of the week is it?, (4) What year is it?, and (5) What time of day is it? (within 1 hour). The number of orientation questions answered correctly determines the orientation score. The immediate memory score captures the athlete's ability to recall five words that are read to them on three separate trials. For example, the athlete is asked to repeat the words: elbow, apple, carpet, saddle, and bubble. The number of words recalled correctly for each trial is then added with a maximum score of 15. Concentration is tested in two parts. Initially, the concussed athlete is read a string of numbers, and then the individual must repeat them in reverse order. For example, the administrator will say: 7-1-9, and the athlete should respond with: 9-1-7. Four trials are completed with number strings of three to six digits long. The second part of concentration testing requires the athlete to recall the months of the year in reverse order. The sum of the correct digits backwards trials and one point for an entirely correct recall of the months in reverse order constitutes the concentration score out of 5.

The SAC can be administered in 5–7 minutes making it a practical sideline assessment tool and athletes suffering from concussion have been shown to have worse scores than baseline and control athletes. However, the SAC presents some shortcomings. First, it only tests a narrow range of neurocognitive functions. It also has a low correlation with other neuropsychological tests, indicating that it is not a comprehensive test [21]. The SAC does not assess brainstem or cerebellar function [9, 22, 23]. Furthermore, athletes are able to memorize sections of the tool via baseline testing or through the experiences of other teammates.

3.2 Balance error scoring system (BESS)

Balance is a complex task that requires intact information from the somatosensory, visual, and vestibular systems as well as an intact central nervous system to maintain a balanced, upright stance [24]. Concussions have been shown to inhibit an individual's ability to appropriately use feedback from the vestibular system when visual and somatosensory inputs are disrupted as a result of traumatic brain injury [25–28]. Therefore, postural stability assessments have also been recognized as an important component of evaluation after concussion [25–28].

The balance error scoring system (BESS) was initially developed as a 3–5 minutes assessment tool used by clinicians for the evaluation of postural stability after a concussion [29]. The BESS consists of 3 three stances: double-leg stance (hands on the hips and feet together), single-leg stance (standing on the non-dominant leg with hands on hips), and a tandem stance (the non-dominant foot is placed behind the dominant foot in a heel-to-toe fashion). The stances are performed on both a firm and foam surface with the eyes closed for 20-second trials. Testers observe the patient or athlete for errors in performance during the balance assessment trials with a maximum of 10 errors for each stance. Types of errors are defined as (1) lifting hands off the iliac crest, (2) opening eyes, (3) stepping, stumbling or falling out of position, (4) abducting the hip by more than 30°, (5) lifting the forefoot or heel, (6) remaining out of the test position in more than 5 seconds [29]. A modified version of the BESS (modified BESS, mBESS) that consists of testing the 3 stances on only a firm surface has even been incorporated into the Sport Concussion Assessment Tool 5 (SCAT 5).

Studies have explored the repeatability and reliability of the BESS. The reliability of this test ranges from poor to good while some studies report reliability coefficients that are below clinically acceptable levels [25, 26, 30]. This wide range of reliability may be due to variability and subjectivity resulting from multiple administrators, therefore, it has been recommended that the same individual administer the BESS for serial testing [25, 26, 30]. Furthermore, studies have recommended that an average of three BESS test administrations be used to improve reliability [25, 26, 30]. Although originally developed as an objective tool, the reliability of BESS can be significantly influenced by the subjective nature of the administrator scoring that athlete. Additionally, further variation is seen among different administrators of the BESS. Likewise, the reliability of the modified BESS is not optimal due to the subjective nature of the scoring system in which the test administrator is required to count errors that include subjective components such as trying to estimate an abduction of the hip by more than 30° or timing a subject out of the testing position by more than 5 seconds. Additionally, low levels of reliability have been reported to be due to subtle changes in balance not detectable by the administrator [25, 26, 30]. Furthermore, stances included in the BESS have been criticized for being either too difficult or too easy for normal healthy controls making it difficult to detect change in performance. In an evaluation of the BESS in a healthy collegiate football cohort at pre-season baseline, the single leg stance accounted for nearly three-quarters of the total errors committed by the study sample. Additionally, over one-fifth of the study participants also demonstrated the maximum error score of 10 errors on the single leg stance. This high variability and large number of errors in the single leg stance leads to concerns over the practical utility of the single leg stance in identifying performance change as a result of suspected concussion [31].

Several other factors are known to influence balance. These include dehydration, ankle bracing, and a prior leg injury [25, 26]. Balance differences have been demonstrated between various training backgrounds and sports played as a result of neuromuscular training. Fatigue following physical exertion has also been shown to adversely affect balance for up to an estimated 20 minutes following physical activity [25, 26]. Therefore, BESS may require a waiting period and should not be successfully administered in 3–5 minutes immediately after the concussive injury.

3.3 Sport concussion assessment tool 5

The SCAT 5 [32] and the Child SCAT 5 [33] are the evaluation tools recommended by the Concussion in Sport Group (CISG) for assessing a suspected concussion. These tests offer a standardized approach to sideline evaluation which incorporates multiple domains of function.

The SCAT 5 for immediate, on-field assessment is comprised of a brief neurological examination which includes an assessment for red flags, observable signs, a brief memory assessment, the Glasgow Coma Scale (GCS) and a cervical spine assessment. Red flags include the following: neck pain or tenderness, double vision, weakness or tingling/burning in arms or legs, severe or increasing headache, seizure or convulsion, loss of consciousness, deteriorating conscious state, vomiting, increasingly restless, agitated or combative. Observable signs are documented as either witnessed or observed on video and include: (1) lying motionless on the playing surface, (2) balance, gait difficulties or motor incoordination: stumbling, slow or labored movements, (3) disorientation or confusion, or an inability to respond appropriately to questions, (4) blank or vacant look, (5) facial injury after head trauma. The brief assessment of memory uses Maddocks questions which include: (1) What venue are we at today? (2) Which half is it now? (3) Who scored last in this match? (4) What team did you play last week or last game? (5) Did your team win the last game? The GCS is scored out of 15 in which an eye, verbal and motor response is evaluated. The best eye response is scored as 1 for no eye opening, 2 for eye opening in response to pain, 3 for eye opening to speech, and 4 eyes opening spontaneously. The best verbal response is scored out of 5 as 1 for no verbal response, 2 for incomprehensible sounds, 3 for inappropriate words, 4 for confused and 5 for oriented. Lastly the best motor response is scored out of 6 as 1 for no motor response, 2 for extension to pain, 3 for abnormal flexion to pain, 4 for flexion or withdrawal to pain, 5 for the ability to localize the pain and 6 for obeying commands. Finally, the cervical spine assessment asks if the athlete reports that their neck is pain free at rest and if so, if there is a full range of active pain free movement. Also, normal limb strength and sensation is evaluated for.

The SCAT 5 in-office or off-field assessment follows the immediate assessment and is comprised of a comprehensive symptom evaluation of 22 symptoms with a 0–5 athlete grading of severity, a brief cognitive assessment using the components of the Standardized Assessment of Concussion (SAC), a neurological screen and a balance assessment using the modified-balance error scoring system.

Changes to the original SAC were made when included in the updated SCAT 5. The SAC immediate memory and delayed recall words lists include an option to use 10 words instead of just 5 in an effort to minimize ceiling effects [32]. Additionally six word lists are presented with alternate stimulus sets for the words list for randomized administration at both baseline and serially during post-injury testing [32]. Similarly, the SAC concentration task of digits backwards in which athletes are asked to repeat back digits in reverse order, contains six versions of the concentration number lists also for randomized use at both baseline and serially during post-injury testing [32]. Additionally, a notation of when the last trial of the word list was administered is required and the delayed recall component of the SAC is recommended to be administered no sooner than 5 minutes following the immediate memory subset.

Although the SCAT 5 tests many cognitive functions related to a concussion, it should be noted that there are some shortcomings. First, it takes 15–20 minutes to complete and must be administered by a medical professional, rendering it inefficient and impractical for sideline evaluation particularly for youth and high school level sports and organizations that do not have access to medical personnel on the sidelines [9]. Additionally as discussed previously, balance performance can be affected by a number of variables and therefore reliability is difficult when attempting to differentiate balance dysfunction as a result of physical fatigue from balance impairment associated with concussion [25, 26]. Therefore, it is recommended that assessment of symptom endorsement and symptom severity, neurocognitive function and balance function take place following a 15-minute rest period to avoid the influence of fatigue or exertion, adding to the time it takes to complete the test following concussive injury [34]. The SCAT symptoms checklist may also be unreliable due to the subjective nature of the evaluation as well as athletes underreporting symptoms to avoid removal from play. Research has indicated that over a quarter of athletes who reported zero symptoms on the checklist still showed cognitive changes following a concussion [35]. In anonymous survey studies of collegiate athletes, nearly half admitted to knowingly hiding symptoms of a concussion to stay in a game and 1 one out of 5 five indicated they would be unlikely or very unlikely to report concussion symptoms to a coach or athletic trainer in the future [23].

3.4 Child sports concussion assessment tool 5

Research has shown that the SCAT testing components are more variable in younger athletes and therefore the Child SCAT 5 is recommended for use by physicians and licensed healthcare professionals in evaluating children aged 5–12 years. In this version, the immediate on-field assessment also includes a check for red flags, observable signs, GCS evaluation and cervical spine assessment.

The Child SCAT 5 in-office or off-field assessment follows the immediate assessment and is comprised of a comprehensive symptom and severity evaluation of 21 symptoms. In this version, symptoms are ranked on a 0–3 scale rather than 0–6, and both children and parents are given a report section in an effort to clear up miscommunication of symptoms. For the concentration component, children are asked to give the days of the week in reverse order, rather than the months in reverse order as asked on the SCAT 5. Additionally, the balance portion of the test is modified to only include the single leg stance in older, 10 through 12-year-old athletes only.

3.5 Concussion recognition tool 5

Although SCAT batteries are to be administered by medical professionals, the Concussion Recognition Tool 5 (CRT 5) was developed for lay person use. The CRT 5 is composed of an assessment for red flags, observable signs, symptoms checklist, and a brief memory assessment [9].

Red flags include the following: neck pain or tenderness, double vision, weakness or tingling/burning in arms or legs, severe or increasing headache, seizure or convulsion, loss of consciousness, deteriorating conscious state, vomiting, increasingly restless, agitated or combative. Observable signs are documented as either witnessed or observed on video and include: (1) lying motionless on the playing surface, (2) disorientation or confusion, or an inability to respond appropriately to questions, (3) balance, gait difficulties or motor incoordination: stumbling, slow or labored movements, (4) slow to get up after a direct or indirect hit to the head, (5) blank or vacant look, (6) facial injury after head trauma. The brief assessment of memory is used only for athletes older than 12 years and includes the following: (1) What venue are we at today? (2) Which half is it now? (3) Who scored last in this match? (4) What team did you play last week or last game? (5) Did your team win the last game? Users are instructed to remove athletes from play if one or more of these indicators are present or if a memory question is answered incorrectly.

3.6 King-Devick test in association with Mayo Clinic

The *King-Devick Test in association with Mayo Clinic* (K-D Test) is a rapid-number naming test used to evaluate for impairments in saccadic eye movements, attention, concentration, and language, which involve integration of functions of the brainstem, cerebellum, and cerebral cortex [36]. The K-D test assesses over half of brain pathways and several cortical areas are involved in saccadic eye movement [36, 37].

The K-D test requires subjects to read a series of 120 single single-digit numbers aloud from left to right across three test screens that progress in difficult as quickly but as accurately as possible. There are several versions of the test to prevent memorization. The total time to complete the test and the errors are recorded. An individualized pre-injury baseline is determined ideal at pre-season and used for comparison during an acute sideline post-injury evaluation. Extensive research has demonstrated worsening in performance in concussed athletes with high sensitivity and specificity [36, 38–41]. A study by the University of Florida found that the K-D test complements components of the SCAT 5, increasing the concussion detection rate in collegiate athletes when using a combination of testing components that include the K-D test, symptoms checklist and balance assessment [38]. Additionally, the K-D test is resistant to the effects of fatigue, showing no worsening of time when athletes were tested in game-like physical fatigue situations [36, 42, 43].

Although athletic trainers or medical professionals are present on the sidelines of professional and collegiate sporting events, most youth and high school sports lack these resources. However, parents, coaches, and laypersons can administer the King-Devick test in less than 2 minutes, making it realistic for sideline concussion evaluation [40, 44, 45].

Multiple studies have also demonstrated the utility of the K-D test in screening for "unwitnessed" concussive events [41, 47–49]. In a large prospective observational cohort study of New Zealand rugby, routine post-match screening was completed with the K-D test and in doing so aiding in identifying 44 unwitnessed, unreported concussions over the duration of the study. This totaled 6 times more than the 8 witnessed concussions, which were identified pitch-side [46]. Researchers reported that by using a composite of rapid brief tests such as the K-D test, the SAC and BESS are likely to provide a series of effective clinical tools to assess players on the sideline with suspected concussive injury [41, 47–49].

4. Clinical management

The majority of sports-related concussion symptoms typically resolve spontaneously within 2 weeks [50]. Younger athletes typically require longer recovery within 4 weeks [51]. The International Concussion in Sport Group currently promotes and supports physical and cognitive rest following concussive injury until acute symptoms resolve [9]. Once symptoms are abated, individuals should then undergo a stepwise, graded program of exertion. Athletes should be symptom free at rest as well as during and after exertion prior to complete medical clearance and full return to play. Recent research supporting the inclusion of active concussion rehabilitation has been reported and may improve outcomes.

4.1 Graduated return to play protocol

The graduated return to play protocol is a stepwise process in which the athlete may continue to proceed to the next level if asymptomatic at the previous level. It is outlined that each step should be 24 hours and therefore the athletes would generally take approximately 1 week to complete all levels of the protocol. If any symptoms arise during any of the levels, the athlete should return to the previous level until asymptomatic and 24 hours of rest has occurred [9, 44].

Rehabilitation stage 1: no activity.
  Symptom limited physical and cognitive rest.
  Objective: recovery.
Rehabilitation stage 2: light aerobic exercise.
  Walking, swimming or stationary cycling keeping intensity <70% maximum permitted heart rate. No resistance training.
  Objective: increase heart rate.
Rehabilitation stage 3: sport-specific exercise.
  Skating drills in ice hockey, running drills in soccer. No head impact activities
  Objective: add movement.
Rehabilitation stage 4: non-contact training drills.
  Progression to more complex training drills (i.e. passing drills in football and ice hockey). May start progressive resistance training.
  Objective: exercise, coordination and cognitive load.
Rehabilitation stage 5: full-contact practice.
  Following medical clearance participate in normal training activities.
  Objective: restore confidence and assess functional skills by coaching staff
Rehabilitation stage 6: return to Play.
  Normal game play

4.2 Active concussion recovery & rehabilitation

Recent research suggests that rest until all symptoms resolve may not be best and that taking a more active approach to recovery for patients with persistent, chronic symptoms may improve recovery outcomes.

Given our understanding of concussion pathophysiology and changes in cerebral blood flow autoregulation as a result of the injury, it is believed that exercise intolerance may be a physiological biomarker of ongoing impairment [52]. Therefore the return of normal exercise tolerance can be then used to establish a sign for physiological recovery from concussion. Using any symptom-exacerbation as an individual's stopping criteria, individualized sub-symptom threshold aerobic exercise treatment programs has been shown to improve recovery time and aerobic ability in athletes with persistent concussion symptoms. This symptom improvement was also associated with improved fitness and autonomic function such as heart rate and blood pressure control and resulted in speeded recovery compared to non-active recovery study participants [53].

Active treatment targeted at system specific deficits that the patient is experiences has been shown to improve recovery. Specifically, ocular motor dysfunction is very common following sports-related concussion with a reported 90% of traumatic brain injury patients reporting vision or visual related symptoms [54]. Symptoms typically include: double vision, blurred vision, headache, dizziness, difficulty with reading or other vision-based tasks. The physical and cognitive control of eye movements requires a majority of the brain's pathways including fronto-parietal, temporal and occipital circuits as well as numerous subcortical nuclei all of which are particularly susceptible to head injury [37]. Several studies have demonstrated the effectivity of ocular based rehabilitation for vision-based deficiencies in the general population and a growing number of investigations are showing similar results in the mTBI population with improvement in vision-related symptoms, reading ability and visual attention [55–58].

5. Conclusion

Given the increasing public awareness and attention revolving sports concussion and the long-term consequences of contact sport and traumatic brain injury exposure, there is growing interest in understanding the complex and concerning issues surrounding sport-related concussion. From what we understand about the pathophysiology of concussion, it is complex and involves a multifactorial process. Many mechanisms that are currently understood from the available literature were described however there is still much more to explore and understand. For example, it is unclear what the role of various factors is in the pathophysiological process. These include the role of genetics, age, gender, premorbid conditions and environmental factors and how they may affect and alter both the underlying pathophysiology, the outward clinical symptomatology experienced by the athlete and the recovery and rehabilitation course of a particular injury. Improved global understanding of these factors will be vital to understanding how best to use an individualized approach to the treatment and management of these patients.

Similarly, the ideal methodology for optimal detection and diagnosis of concussion is multifaceted requiring the use of a suite of tools to evaluate multiple systems. In the acute setting it is highly important that these assessments be quick, efficient and accurate in detecting deficits in performance that are associated with concussion. Likewise, these evaluations need to be able to be practically implemented on the sidelines therefore cost and efficient are heavily weighted. Simultaneously, concussion awareness by all stakeholders will aid in improving outcomes from this injury. Athletes, coaches, officials and other stakeholders need to be educated on the signs and symptoms of concussion, the long-term risks of continuing to participate in sports activity with a brain injury and therefore the importance of timely removal from play as well as the equally imperativeness of appropriate clearance for return to play.

Rehabilitation of sports-related concussion is ever changing given continued ongoing research which gives insights into the latest and best recommended approaches to caring and managing patients during their recovery to improve overall outcomes. The current method is a targeted and individualized approach. Additionally, active rehabilitation has been shown to be beneficial, particularly in patients with extended recovery durations and prolonged symptomatology. Continued investigations will help answer the questions of how treatments should vary among individuals based on their makeup, for example, their concussion history, outset signs and symptoms, as well as children vs. adults. These likely all play a role and can assist in developing more targeted rehabilitation programs for individuals to advance therapies.

Conflict of interest

Dr. Leong is employed by King-Devick technologies, Inc. as Chief Scientific Officer.

Author details

Danielle Leong[1,2]

1 King-Devick Technologies, Inc., Oakbrook Terrace, IL, USA

2 Illinois Eye Institute, Chicago, IL, USA

*Address all correspondence to: danielle.leong@kingdevick.com

References

[1] Hilgers L. Youth Sports Drawing more than Ever [Internet]. 2006. Available from: http://www.cnn.com/2006/US/07/03/rise.kids.sports/

[2] Centers for Disease Control and Prevention. Nonfatal traumatic brain injuries related to sports and recreation activities among persons aged </=19 years-United States, 2001-2009. Morbidity and Mortality Weekly Report. 2011;**60**(39):1337-1342

[3] Langlois JA, Rutland-Brown W, Wald MM. The epidemiology and impact of traumatic brain injury: A brief overview. The Journal of Head Trauma Rehabilitation. 2006;**21**(5):375-378

[4] Ferguson R. Game Changers: Stats, Stories and What Communities Are Doing to Protect Young Athletes [Internet]. Safe Kids Worldwide Anlaysis of CPSC NEISS Data. 2013. Available from: https://www.safekids.org/sites/default/files/documents/ResearchReports/final_sports_study_2013.pdf

[5] Bakhos LL, Lockhart GR, Myers R, Linakis JG. Emergency department visits for concussion in young child athletes. Pediatrics. 2010;**126**(16):e550-e556

[6] American Association of Neurological Surgeons. Sports-Related Head Injury [Internet]. 2011. Available from: https://www.aans.org/Patients/Neurosurgical-Conditions-and-Treatments/Sports-related-Head-Injury

[7] Marar M, McIlvain NM, Fields SK, Comstock RD. Epidemiology of concussions among United States high school athletes in 20 sports. The American Journal of Sports Medicine. 2012;**40**:747-755

[8] McCrea M, Hammeke T, Olsen G, Leo P, Guskiewicz K. Unreported concussion in high school football players: Implications for prevention. Clinical Journal of Sport Medicine. 2004;**14**(1):13-17

[9] McCrory P, Meeuwisse WH, Aubry M, Cantu RC, Dvorák J, Echemendia RJ, et al. Consensus statement on concussion in sport-the 4th international conference on concussion in sport held in Zurich, November 2012. PM & R: The Journal of Injury, Function, and Rehabilitation. 2013;**5**:255-279

[10] Dziemianowicz MS, Kirschen MP, Pukenas BA, Laudano E, Balcer LJ, Galetta SL. Sports-related concussion testing. Current Neurology and Neuroscience Reports. 2012;**12**(5):547-559

[11] Plassman BL, Havlik RJ, Steffens DC, Helms MJ, Newman TN, Drosdick D, et al. Documented head injury in early adulthood and risk of Alzheimer's disease and other dementias. Neurology. 2000;**55**(8):1158-1166

[12] Stern RA, Riley DO, Daneshvar DH, Nowinski CJ, Cantu RC, McKee AC. Long-term consequences of repetitive brain trauma: Chronic traumatic encephalopathy. PM & R: The Journal of Injury, Function, and Rehabilitation. 2011;**3**(October):460-467

[13] McKee AC, Stein TD, Nowinski CJ, Stern RA, Daneshvar DH, Alvarez VE, et al. The spectrum of disease in chronic traumatic encephalopathy. Brain. 2013;**136**:43-64

[14] Gavett BE, Stern RA, Cantu RC, Nowinski CJ, AC MK. Mild traumatic brain injury: A risk factor for neurodegeneration. Alzheimer's Research & Therapy. 2010;**2**:18

[15] McKee AC, Daneshvar DH, Alvarez VE, Stein TD. The neuropathology of sport. Acta Neuropathologica. 2014;**127**(1):29-51

[16] Meaney DF, Smith DH. Concussion in sports biomechanics of concussion. Clinics in Sports Medicine. 2014;**30**(1):19-31. DOI: 10.1016/j.csm.2010.08.009

[17] Steenerson K, Starling A. Pathophysiology of sports-related concussion concussion. Neurologic Clinics. 2017;**35**(3):403-408. DOI: 10.1016/j.ncl.2017.03.011

[18] Choe MC. The pathophysiology of concussion. Current Pain and Headache Reports. 2016;**20**(6):42. DOI: 10.1007/s11916-016-0573-9

[19] Dixon KJ. Pathophysiology of traumatic B rain injury. Physical Medicine and Rehabilitation Clinics of North America. 2019;**28**(2):215-225. DOI: 10.1016/j.pmr.2016.12.001

[20] Goldstein LE, Fisher AM, Tagge CA, Zhang X-L, Velisek L, Sullivan JA, et al. Chronic traumatic encephalopathy in blast-exposed military veterans and a blast neurotrauma mouse model. Science Translational Medicine. 2012;**4**:134-160

[21] Broglio SP, Schnebel B, Sosnoff JJ, Shin S, Feng X, He X, et al. Biomechanical properties of concussions in high school football. Medicine and Science in Sports and Exercise. 2010;**42**(11):2064-2071

[22] McCrory P, Meeuwisse W, Johnston K, Dvorak J, Aubry M, Molloy M, et al. Consensus statement on concussion in sport: The 3rd international conference on concussion in sport held in Zurich, November 2008. Journal of Athletic Training. 2009;**44**(4):434-448

[23] Torres DM, Galetta KM, Phillips HW, Dziemianowicz EMS, Wilson JA, Dorman ES, et al. Sports-related concussion anonymous survey of a collegiate cohort. Neurology Clinical Practice. 2013;**3**(August):279-287

[24] Diener HC, Dichgans J, Guschlbauer B, Bacher M. Role of visual and static vestibular influences on dynamic posture control. Human Neurobiology. 1986;**5**(2):105-113

[25] Hunt TN, Ferrara MS, Bornstein RA, Baumgartner TA. The reliability of the modified balance error scoring system. Clinical Journal of Sport Medicine. 2009;**19**(6):471-475

[26] Bell DR, Guskiewicz KM, Clark MA, Padua DA. Systematic review of the balance error scoring system. Sports Health: A Multidisciplinary Approach. 2011;**3**(3):287-295

[27] Guskiewicz KM, Broglio SP. Sport-related concussion: On-field and sideline assessment. Physical Medicine and Rehabilitation Clinics of North America. 2011;**22**:603-617

[28] Guskiewicz KM. Assessment of postural stability following sport-related concussion. Current Sports Medicine Reports. 2003;**2**:24-30

[29] Guskiewicz KM, Ross SE, Marshall SW. Postural stability and neuropsychological de cits after concussion in collegiate athletes. Journal of Athletic Training. 2001;**36**(3):263-273

[30] Guskiewicz KM. Balance assessment in the management of sport-related concussion. Clinics in Sports Medicine. 2011;**30**(1):89-102.ix

[31] Starling A, Leong D, Bogle J, Vargas B. Variability of the modified balance error scoring system at baseline using objective and subjective balance measures. Concussion. 2015;**1**(1):CNC5

[32] Echemendia RJ, Meeuwisse W, McCrory P, Davis GA, Putukian M, Leddy J, et al. The sport concussion assessment tool 5th edition (SCAT5): Background and rationale. British Journal of Sports Medicine. 2017;**51**(11):848-850

[33] Davis GA, Purcell L, Schneider KJ, Yeates KO, Gioia GA, Anderson V, et al. The child sport concussion assessment tool 5th edition (child SCAT5): Background and rationale. British Journal of Sports Medicine. 2017;**51**(11): 859-861

[34] Guskiewicz KM, Register-Mihalik J, McCrory P, McCrea M, Johnston K, Makdissi M, et al. Evidence-based approach to revising the SCAT2: Introducing the SCAT3. British Journal of Sports Medicine. 2013;**47**:289-293

[35] Kriz PK, Mannix R, Taylor AM, Ruggieri D, Meehan WP. Neurocognitive deficits of concussed adolescent athletes in self-reported symptom resolution in the zurich guidelines era. Orthopaedic Journal of Sports Medicine. 2017;**5**(11):2325967117737307

[36] Galetta K, Liu M, Leong DF, Ventura RE, Galetta S, Balcer L. The King-Devick test of rapid number naming for concussion detection: Meta-analysis and systematic review of the literature. Concussion. 2015;**1**(2):CNC8. DOI: 10.2217/cnc.15.8

[37] Ventura RE, Balcer LJ, Galetta SL. The neuro-ophthalmology of head trauma. Lancet Neurology. 2014;**13**(10):1006-1016. DOI: 10.1016/S1474-4422(14)70111-5

[38] Marinides Z, Galetta KM, Andrews CN, Wilson JA, Herman DC, Robinson CD, et al. Vision testing is additive to the sideline assessment of sports-related concussion. Neurology Clinical Practice. 2014;**5**(1):25-34

[39] Dhawan P, Starling A, Tapsell L, Adler J, Galetta S, Balcer L, et al. King-Devick test identifies symptomatic concussion in real-time and asymptomatic concussion over time. Neurology. 2014;**82**(10_Supplement):S11.003

[40] Leong DF, Balcer LJ, Galetta SL, Liu Z, Master CL. The King-Devick test as a concussion screening tool administered by sports parents. The Journal of Sports Medicine and Physical Fitness. 2013;**54**(February):70-77

[41] King D, Brughelli M, Hume P, Gissane C. Concussions in amateur rugby union identified with the use of a rapid visual screening tool. Journal of the Neurological Sciences. 2013;**326**: 59-63. DOI: 10.1016/j.jns.2013.01.012

[42] Galetta KM, Brandes LE, Maki K, Dziemianowicz MS, Laudano E, Allen M, et al. The King-Devick test and sports-related concussion: Study of a rapid visual screening tool in a collegiate cohort. Journal of the Neurological Sciences. 2011;**309**:34-39. DOI: 10.1016/j.jns.2011.07.039

[43] Leong DF, Balcer LJ, Galetta SL, Evans G, Gimre M, Watt D. The King-Devick test for sideline concussion screening in collegiate football. Journal of Optometry. 2015;**8**(2):131-139

[44] Harmon KG, Drezner JA, Gammons M, Guskiewicz KM, Halstead M, Herring SA, et al. American medical Society for sports medicine position statement: Concussion in sport. British Journal of Sports Medicine. 2013;**47**:15-26

[45] Silver D, Brown N, Gissane C. Reported concussion incidence in youth community Rugby union and parental assessment of post head injury cognitive recovery using the King-Devick test. Journal of the Neurological Sciences. 2018;**388**:40-46. DOI: 10.1016/j.jns.2018.02.046

[46] King D, Hume P, Gissane C, Clark T. Use of the King-Devick test for sideline concussion screening in junior rugby league. Journal of the Neurological Sciences. 2015;**357**(1-2):75-79

[47] King D, Clark T, Gissane C. Use of a rapid visual screening tool for the assessment of concussion in amateur rugby league: A pilot study. Journal of the Neurological Sciences. 2012;**320** (1-2):16-21. DOI: 10.1016/j.jns.2012.05.049

[48] King D, Gissane C, Hume PA, Flaws M. The King-Devick test was useful in management of concussion in amateur rugby union and rugby league in New Zealand. Journal of the Neurological Sciences. 2015;**351**:58-64

[49] Hecimovich M, King D, Dempsey AR, Murphy M. The King-Devick test is a valid and reliable tool for assessing sport-related concussion in Australian football: A prospective cohort study. Journal of Science and Medicine in Sport. 2018;**21**(10):1004-1007. DOI: 10.1016/j.jsams.2018.03.011

[50] McCrea M, Guskiewicz K, Randolph C, Barr WB, Hammeke TA, Marshall SW, et al. Incidence, clinical course, and predictors of prolonged recovery time following sport-related concussion in high school and college athletes. Journal of the International Neuropsychological Society. 2013;**19**(1):22-33

[51] Zemek R, Barrowman N, Freedman SB, Gravel J, Gagnon I, McGahern C, et al. Clinical risk score for persistent postconcussion symptoms among children with acute concussion in the ED. Journal of the American Medical Association. 2016;**315**(10):1014-1025

[52] Darling SR, Leddy JJ, Baker JG, Williams AJ, Surace A, Miecznikowski JC, et al. Evaluation of the Zurich guidelines and exercise testing for return to play in adolescents following concussion. Clinical Journal of Sport Medicine: Official Journal of the Canadian Academy of Sport Medicine. 2014;**24**(2):128-133

[53] Leddy JJ, Kozlowski K, Donnelly JP, Pendergast DR, Epstein LH, Willer B. A preliminary study of subsymptom threshold exercise training for refractory post-concussion syndrome. Clinical Journal of Sport Medicine. 2010;**20**(1):21-27

[54] Ciuffreda KJ, Kapoor N, Rutner D, Suchoff IB, Han ME, Craig S. Occurrence of oculomotor dysfunctions in acquired brain injury: A retrospective analysis. Optometry. 2007;**78**:155-161

[55] Thiagarajan P, Ciuffreda KJ. Effect of oculomotor rehabilitation on vergence responsivity in mild traumatic brain injury. Journal of Rehabilitation Research and Development. 2014;**50**(7):1223-1240

[56] Yadav NK, Thiagarajan P, Ciuffreda KJ. Effect of oculomotor vision rehabilitation on the visual-evoked potential and visual attention in mild traumatic brain injury. Brain Injury. 2014;**28**(7):922-929

[57] Thiagaragjan P, Ciuffreda K. Versional eye tracking in mild traumatic brain injury (mTBI): Effects of oculomotor training. Brain Injury. 2014;**28**(7):930-943

[58] Thiagarajan P, Ciuffreda KJ, Capo-Aponte JE, Ludlam DP, Kapoor N. Oculomotor neurorehabilitation for reading in mild traumatic brain injury (mTBI): An integrative approach. NeuroRehabilitation. 2014;**34**:129-146

Chapter 2

The Primary Care Sports and Exercise Medicine Physician: A Key Role in a Continuum Remodeling Medical Career

Felipe Hardt and Rafael Cristiano Geiss Santos

Abstract

The characteristics of the primary care sports and exercise medicine physicians (SEMP) have been evolving over the past decades. Nowadays, the sports medicine physician is a highly qualified professional, with a slightly different spectrum of training background according to which part of the globe he/she specialized. Uniquely trained to provide care along the continuum of injuries and illnesses, from the acute evaluation to return to sport, to manage complications and coexisting medical issues, the SEMP are in a critical position to provide a comprehensive management plan to optimize health and performance for the athletes and to develop healthy lifestyles by counseling on physical activity and exercise within the healthcare system. The objective of this chapter is to provide the readers a general overview of the SEMP training, the skills and abilities the primary care physician must pursuit and qualify, and its role from recreational sports to elite level and as a healthy lifestyle promoter.

Keywords: primary care, sports and exercise medicine, health promotion, physical activity, athlete, performance

1. The primary care sports and exercise medicine physician: overview, characteristics, and particularities

In the past, sports medicine has been understood of as a medical field solely related to the elite, professional, or Olympic competitive athletes and not accessible for the regular person. Lately, sports medicine has grown from a special interest area in healthcare to an established profession in the medical career [1, 2].

Currently, sports medicine might be defined as the medical specialty concerned with the care and well-being of athletes and those engaged in physical activity, working as a health manager providing a comprehensive management plan to optimize health and performance for the athletes and to develop healthy lifestyles by counseling on physical activity and exercise within the healthcare system [1–4].

The specialty as a primary care field encompasses many different disciplines and areas of expertise, such as internal medicine, family medicine, orthopedics, exercise science, cardiology, neurology, pediatrics, and emergency medicine. Sports medicine physicians, with their focus on sports and exercise medicine, are uniquely trained to provide such expertise to patients and medical colleagues [3, 5].

As consultants, they can be of great help in evaluating and treating active patients by efficiently connecting the different medical fields. Primary care sports medicine physicians can facilitate early diagnosis and management, thus accelerating recovery and avoiding long-term disability, providing adequate management, and eliminating the need for further consultation.

Patients can be seen quickly and cost-effectively. Therefore, sports doctors can reduce long waiting lists, solve the shortage of other specialists, and reduce the rising costs of healthcare. There is clearly an important role for the knowledge of sports medicine in the integral care of patients [1, 6].

However, the specialist physician in sports medicine is not always well understood by fellow doctors, health workers, team managers, and politicians. It is very challenging to change the current paradigms based on existing diseases in the health systems and the beliefs of the population, where the pharmaceutical industry has significant financial and political influence.

A consistent, sustained, and coordinated effort by the wider medical community, aligned with a bold political vision to change health systems and society's culture to promote and support physical activity, is a crucial requirement.

2. A general overview of the SEMP training and medical background

2.1 Undergraduate training

As a general overview, medical students usually do not have many learning opportunities in sports medicine during regular medical programs. Previous publications evidenced that medical students would favor having more exposure to sports and exercise medicine and even suggest compulsory sports medicine education. Similarly, general practitioners feel inadequately trained to practice sports and exercise medicine [7–11].

Besides this hidden barrier, sports medicine is being more recognized as a potentially attractive career to be pursued by a growing number of young doctors all over the world. Sports and exercise medicine is a multidisciplinary specialty, which has the potential to provide a medical student with valuable learning opportunities at various stages of his/her training [1, 9, 12].

An increase in demand for sports medicine training would facilitate on understanding the specific field, its demands, and possible career pathways for the graduating physician. Program directors of the universities and medical schools should include sports and exercise medicine in their curricula and use the expertise of sports medicine physicians in their community. Lectures and clinical skill workshops on sports-related illness, injuries, and musculoskeletal examination should be included in the undergraduate years, complemented later by electives and rotations in sports medicine [7, 9].

2.2 Postgraduate training

The profession is moving firmly from the previous concept of "athlete's medicine" toward a vision where the main concern of specialists is physical activity promotion. The current definition of sports and exercise medicine can be extended to public health, presenting greater impact on improving the overall health of the population and assisting the expansion of the specialty [1, 4, 12–14].

A high-quality structured education in the field of sports and exercise medicine should be the critical goal for practicing physicians. Primary care sports medicine fellowship programs are designed to provide comprehensive training in preventing and treating musculoskeletal and non-musculoskeletal conditions in athletes and active individuals [3].

The specific pathways and entrance criteria for the specialty might be slightly different depending on the country and medical boards. Although most of the programs have their organization and structure, there are no universal criteria established to describe benchmarks for quality improvement or standards of excellence. Every program has its specific strengths [5, 12, 15].

For instance, primary care sports medicine physicians in Canada and the United States follow a 1-year specialized fellowship training program. Practitioners can enter these programs via many routes, including other specialties, such as internal medicine, pediatrics, emergency medicine, physical medicine, and rehabilitation [3, 5].

On the other hand, New Zealand, Australia, and Brazil have similar training criteria, as do many European nations. In those countries, physicians can pursue the sports medicine residency as a 3–4-year program, immediately after graduating from medical school [5, 12, 15].

The sports medicine programs must provide specific areas of knowledge to properly qualify the sports medicine physician, as quality education should be the goal of all fellowship/residency programs. All sports medicine physicians must have comprehensive training in preventing and treating musculoskeletal and non-musculoskeletal conditions in athletes and active individuals [3, 5, 12].

Fellowships and residencies usually include training areas of internal medicine, pediatrics, clinical emergencies across the lifespan, rehabilitation, physiatry, orthopedics, exercise physiology, cardiology, pulmonology, rheumatology, and sports nutrition and practical training in events, clubs, specific sports, general exercise, and sports medicine care. Programs must also include theoretical education, including organizing/leading discussions, seminars, and clinical case reviews and attending lectures and medical ethics courses [3, 5, 12].

3. Sports and exercise medicine physician-specific training, skills, and abilities

This section does not intend to determine the specific contents of the sports medicine programs. Its purpose is to demonstrate some of the core competencies of the sports medicine training and to provide additional information for the physician with interest in the specific field of practice [3, 5, 12].

4. Essential competencies

4.1 Patient care and medical knowledge

The primary care sports and exercise medicine fellow/resident must be trained inpatient care to be able to diagnose and provide treatment of medical illnesses and injuries related to sports and exercise and proficiently perform all procedures essential to the practice of sports medicine. Medical development must include also biomedical, epidemiological, and social/behavioral sciences and its application to patient care [3, 5, 12].

The training doctor must be exposed to a different setting and clinical situations, with broad clinical experience, high patient load, and follow-ups, including different age groups, sports, genders, socioeconomic levels, types of sports, and levels of participation.

4.2 Event coverage

Fellows/residents should be exposed to event coverage in a variety of settings during their training year(s). These include covering youth or senior/professional sports teams; participating in elite-level Olympic sports, such as athletics, swimming, and gymnastics; and coverage of mass events, such as marathon or triathlon major events.

It is extremely important to participate in a variety of sports to become accustomed to the athletic environment and potential injuries that could be sustained during the events, possibly including coverage to contact sports to be exposed to concussion and other contact injuries.

4.3 Pre-participation examination (PPE)

Programs of excellence will have training doctors to perform pre-participation examinations for a variety of athletes and disciplines, including team sports, individual sports, elite, and young athletes.

4.4 Specialty and orthopedics rotations

Residents/fellows rotate with subspecialists; including sports cardiology; musculoskeletal radiology; rehabilitation; physical/occupational therapy; exercise physiology and performance; neurology; rheumatology; nutrition; psychology; orthopedic surgeons of shoulder, elbow, wrist/hand, hip, knee, and foot/ankle; and pediatric surgeons.

4.5 Acute injury and fracture management

This provides exposure to acute fracture and dislocation management including assessment and diagnosis, splinting and casting.

4.6 ECG interpretation and exercise testing

These include training about the specific adaptations in the athlete's heart, normal changes and pathological abnormalities. These perform and interpret the exams, provide proper care, and identify the need for continued investigations and referrals as needed.

4.7 Exercise prescription

Training on exercise prescription in the different population, their requirements, and specific needs.

4.8 Sports medicine procedures and sports ultrasound

Regarding this specific topic, there might be differences between programs and learning experiences, according to the country and expected field of work. In our understanding, these procedures are an integral component of most sports medicine practices and will be mentioned here.

Injections and other procedures to consider for general exposure include dry needling, autologous blood injections, platelet-rich plasma injections, and prolotherapy. Procedural training should include education in didactic theoretical and practical sessions, including mentored clinical experience and continuing education options to determine proficiency for all procedures.

Sports ultrasound might also be included in the training programs and is seen as an important skill to be performed. Current endorsements for recommended sports ultrasound curriculum for sports and exercise medicine physicians can be found in published journals and sports medicine associations [16].

4.9 Interpersonal skills and communication

Ability to work in a multidisciplinary team and to communicate efficiently are extremely important for the proper patient care not only in a team environment as a team doctor but also for best of care in the outpatient care directing proper multi-professional and teamwork for the patients.

5. The sports and exercise medicine physician medical role: from elite sports and events to healthy lifestyle promoter

The broad and specific knowledge of SEMP, when following a proper training program, allows him/her to provide comprehensive care of patients, being able to handle most of the illnesses and injuries, from the pre-participation assessment to the return-to-play decision.

The primary care sports medicine physicians can facilitate early diagnosis and management, thereby speeding recovery and preventing long-term disability. The appropriate case management, either with physiotherapy, bracing, and orthotics, injections, can optimize treatment pathways, eliminate the need for further consultation, and save time and healthcare costs.

The role of the specialist sports medicine physician is not always well-understood by medical colleagues, team managers, healthcare directors, and politicians. We here describe some of the characteristics of the sports doctor in the elite athlete care approach, event coverage, and healthy lifestyle promotion, including some interprofessional relationships needed in this field, which are usually different from regular working relations and organization found in the more traditional medical specialties.

5.1 Sports and exercise medicine in the elite level

The team physician's education, training, and experience uniquely qualify to provide the best medical care for the athlete. Team physicians have the leadership role in the organization, management, and provision of care of athletes in individual, team, and mass participation sporting events.

The team physician should possess, be responsible for, and/or understand not only clinical illness and injuries, but also medical and administrative duties, ethical matters, medicolegal problems. This role must be developed to provide a foundation for best practices in the medical care of athletes and teams. The most important responsibility is the medical care of athletes at all ages and all levels of participation [17].

The team physician should be proficient in the prevention and care of musculoskeletal injuries and medical conditions encountered in sports. The team physician integrates medical expertise with medical consultants, strength and conditioning coaches, and other allied healthcare professionals. The team physician also is responsible for educating athletes, coaches, parents, and administrators. The team physician is ultimately responsible for the clearance to participate and the return-to-play decision [17, 18].

Expected requirements for the team physician are clinical training and experience including medical specialty board certification, residency/fellowship training in sports medicine, significant clinical practice focused on sports medicine, strong ethical values, proper management of confidentiality issues, informed consent, conflict of interest, influence of third parties, doping, drugs, sports products, and technology [17, 18].

The primary role of the sports medicine physician in competitive sports is the comprehensive health management of the athlete to optimize performance. Sports medicine physicians should focus on providing continuous clinical services with excellence, always in conjunct work with the coach and other members of the sports medicine and science team [13].

In this role, the sports medicine physician is involved in the rehabilitation of acute and chronic injuries as well as developing measures to reduce the risk of injury and illness occurrence or severity. To fulfill this role of comprehensive health management and athletes' performance, the sports medicine physician must understand the demands and requirements of the athlete's sports thoroughly.

An important part of elite sports physician role is the periodic health evaluation, which is the systematic evaluation of the health status of the athlete, seeking the best healthcare but also finding opportunities to optimize the athlete's performance. These must be managed as a health assessment plan, based on initial assessments, follow-ups, and continued care, including cardiovascular screening, general health, clinical laboratory investigation (pertinent lab tests according to sports or discipline), and previous health information [13, 17–19].

The sports physician is the best person from medical staff to coordinate and manage a comprehensive illness and injury plan for elite athletes following that. The combination of excellence in clinical skills, sports-specific knowledge, and a thorough understanding of the athlete's goal will make the sports medicine physician a trusted and respected member of the athlete support team.

The physician work environment might be different from the regular clinical office in the hospital as seen during the medical school. It might vary from a sports medicine institute to a training venue, sideline stretcher, or even a hotel room. It is important to be organized and to be able to record all medical information for proper medical care. Be fully aware that not always there will be a computer or a proper way to document the medical information. Improvisation is a key ability for the sports physician.

Therefore, appropriate clinical communication strategies will facilitate these situations. Multidisciplinary and integrated healthcare is a must for the elite athlete. Efficient and direct communication involving the athlete, coach, and members of the healthcare team are key elements to succeed in this environment [2, 20, 21].

In this perspective, another key point is to develop a clear risk decision-making strategy for the difficult situations involving the athlete's health, specific clinical conditions (illness or injuries), competitions, and the athlete's career. The role of the sports medicine physician is to present clear and precise information to the coach, pertinent staff, and athlete regarding the nature of the injury, possible interventions, the expected rehabilitation course and the timeframe to return to play, and, more importantly, the consequences of continuing to train or compete while injured [20, 21].

Having good relationships and proper understanding of the sports and integration within the team, the sports medicine physician can guide an appropriate path in these challenging circumstances. When working within clubs and organizations, it is ideal if the chief sports medicine physician and the head coach are also aligned with the performance team and the board of directors [2, 22].

Life-threatening emergency situations or conditions in which the athlete is not capable of taking decisions properly do not fit in this process. In these cases, the final decision must be clearly medical to guarantee the physical integrity and life of the athlete.

Besides, the role of sports medicine physicians in optimizing health and performance must be clearly defined and set apart from the malicious practice of doping in sports. It is a fundamental part of the job to educate the athletes, coaches, and managers about clean sports practice, the need for continued surveillance and health and career implications of doping medications and methods.

The sports medicine field demands effective collaboration between the respective disciplines and professions. It requires cooperation between different practitioners (physicians, physiotherapists, athletic trainers) to provide the care required by top-level performing athletes [2, 22].

The essential multidisciplinary nature of the field makes it difficult to define a medical specialty niche. There is a frequent overlapping nature of these professionals and disciplines, making difficult to define the identity of the sports physician. Thus, clear communication policies must be established and followed to avoid problematic issues between contribution and professional boundaries [2].

Unlike conventional health services, where physicians have a very visible professional status, in sports medicine, this status must be granted by relevant athletic experience. Also, some resistance to collaboration may come from a combination of doubt from a professional who comes from outside the sports networks established long ago in the team and an immediate assumption from the doctor that he or she will be effortlessly integrated into it [2].

While there are inevitably tensions surrounding traditional hierarchies, a system that encourages regular professional contact, as well as interprofessional learning opportunities, can gradually reverse these perceptions.

The team doctor role is based on clinical competencies, including pre-participation in health evaluations, integrated medical records, health and performance-focused risk decision-making, integration of communication, and implementation strategies within the specific sport. All of these are applied in a very close relation to the athlete, coach, and staff in a collaborative, balanced, evidence, and preference-based, individualized approach.

5.2 Sports events direction and coordination

The sports medicine physician has an exclusive and important role in the major sports events, such as Olympic Games, Youth Olympic Games, The Fédération Internationale de Football Association (FIFA) World Cup, and world-level competitions. The unique know-how of the daily needs of the athletes, coaches, and specific disciplines or sports, in addition to the people management skills required by the daily sports medicine routine, makes the experienced sports medicine physician a key role in the successful organization and leadership of the major sports events.

The role includes organizing and planning medical care for players, team officials, event officials, and staff; doping control; management of healthcare issues; coordination with local organizing medical services; and injury assessment. The role requires exhaustive programming to preserve the athlete's health and to optimize all collaborative work with individual sports governing bodies. It is part of the sports medicine physician responsibility to create plans for medical emergency responses, staff education, staff selection, background checks, medical equipment, and medication requirements for the specific event [13, 18, 23, 24].

5.3 The sports and exercise medicine physician as healthy lifestyle promoter

Physical inactivity is a huge contributor to global health and a persistent public health problem associated with cardiovascular disease (CVD) and another noncommunicable disease. The World Health Organization ranks it as the fourth leading risk factor for overall morbidity and mortality worldwide [1, 25–27].

Inadequate physical activity is related to a considerable economic burden, and reports indicate that one third of the global population fails to meet physical activity (PA) guidelines and that 9% of the overall global premature mortality, 5.3 million deaths, is directly attributable to physical inactivity [4, 6, 25–28].

As a result, there has been a significant growing global campaign on sports and exercise as key elements to address this pandemic by organizations such as the World Health Organization, International Olympic Committee, and Sports and Exercise Medical Societies promoting physical activity programs in the population [4, 6, 14, 25–29].

The health and economic burden related to the sedentary lifestyle urges the importance of combating physical inactivity. There is substantial evidence to support the benefits of exercise and the cost-effectiveness of exercise prescription in primary care [1, 6, 27, 30–32].

Sports medicine physicians play an important role in the dissemination of exercise recommendations to a great segment of the population. Due to the specialization in restoring function, combined with the background of team-based care in sports medicine, sports physicians are in a unique position to expand their scope of practice to use the expertise in promoting exercise in the community. It is the sports physician role to be proactive in counseling patients for prevention and treatment of such a sedentary lifestyle and its related diseases [1, 4].

Improving and maintaining recommended levels of physical activity lead to reductions in metabolic, hemodynamic, body composition, and risk factors that contribute strongly to the development of many of the major noncommunicable diseases. Therefore, exercise has a significant role, in many cases comparable or superior to drug interventions, in its prevention and management [1, 4, 30, 33].

Similarly, studies show that exercise interventions might be more effective than drug treatment among patients with stroke and as effective as medications for the prevention of diabetes and secondary treatment of cardiovascular disease. Physical activity can be as effective as medications for the treatment of depression and cognitive function in patients with Alzheimer disease [27].

Several high-level systematic reviews have also identified risk reductions of 25–50% or more in most major chronic diseases for individuals who achieve 150 min of moderate to vigorous physical activity per week. Although this target of 150 min may seem out of reach for many who are sedentary, studies have shown significant benefits for those who complete even small amounts of physical activity [27, 30, 34].

The sports and exercise medicine physician should have a key role in the promotion, integration, and facilitation of exercise as medicine within the healthcare system. Sports medicine physicians, with their focus on sports and exercise medicine, are uniquely trained to provide such expertise to patients, learners, and other physicians [1].

Helping patients to move from being sedentary to engaging in moderate levels of physical activity significantly reduces the risk of mortality. The medical specialist closest to the integration of exercise and health are sports and exercise medicine physicians, promoting comprehensive lifestyle interventions to patients for the prevention and management of chronic disease, along with expertise in the evaluation and management of medical conditions affecting activity and sports.

Evidence supporting the health benefits of physical activity is undeniable, and there is strong evidence that physicians can influence patients to significantly improve their health through proactive recommendations on the positive impacts of exercise on health during an office visit. Simple actions such as written exercise prescription, counseling and telephone support, or having the patient to wear a pedometer have a significant influence on engaging patients to be more active and healthy [1, 29, 35–37].

However, the sports medicine physician must be aware of barriers to overcome toward the healthy lifestyle promotion. These include the absence of structured systems to offer to counsel, including the limited staff, insufficient time to provide proper counseling services, and patient care primarily focused on acute care or problem-based care, rather than on preventive care or health promotion. Ameliorating population levels of physical activity require comprehensive efforts under a coordinated multilevel approach [1, 6, 26, 29].

Different strategies might be necessary to overcome the current barriers and provide efficient patient care as a general health manager. The sports physician must assess individual needs; address individual motivation, habits, preferences, and barriers; establish clear and realistic goals; promote behavioral change approaches; and establish follow-up, self-monitoring, and social support. Wearable technology and mobile apps for exercise monitoring might be also a very helpful strategy [33, 36].

Longitudinal follow-up is crucial to determine the patient's progress, address specific problems, identify needs, and even adjust goals. Doctors should assess the physical activity level at each office visit. Also, establishing networks for exercise programs to standardize exercise interventions for different clinical subpopulations and to accommodate the continuum of primordial to tertiary prevention programs are very important. Studies have shown that physician counseling and exercise referral systems promote improvements in patients' physical activity levels for up to 12 months.

6. Conclusion

Primary care sports medicine is a growing field in which the physician is trained exclusively to provide care throughout the continuum of injuries and illnesses, from acute assessment to return to sport, to managing complications and coexisting medical problems.

Sports medicine physicians are in a critical position to provide a comprehensive management plan to optimize athletes' health and performance and to develop healthy lifestyles by advising them on physical activities and exercises in the health system.

The broad and specific knowledge provides comprehensive assistance to patients, being able to deal with most illnesses and injuries, from the pre-participation evaluation to the return-to-play decision. Sports physicians can facilitate early diagnosis and management of illness and injuries, accelerate recovery and avoid long-term disability, provide adequate management, and eliminate the need for further consultation.

The field of sports medicine requires effective collaboration between their respective disciplines and professions, whether as a team physician, event coordinator, or as a health manager promoting a healthy lifestyle.

Author details

Felipe Hardt[1*] and Rafael Cristiano Geiss Santos[2]

1 Department of Sport, School of Physical Education and Sport University of São Paulo, São Paulo, Brazil

2 Sports Medicine Department, Aspetar Orthopaedic and Sports Medicine Hospital, Doha, Qatar

*Address all correspondence to: hardt@usp.br

References

[1] Joy E, Blair SN, McBride P, Sallis R. Physical activity counselling in sports medicine: A call to action. British Journal of Sports Medicine. 2013;**47**(1):49-53. DOI: 10.1136/bjsports-2012-091620

[2] Fletcher S, Breitbach AP, Reeves S. Interprofessional collaboration in sports medicine: Findings from a scoping review. Health & Interprofessional Practice. 2017;**3**:eP1128. DOI: 10.7710/2159-1253.1128

[3] Asif IM, Stovak M, Ray T, Weiss-Kelly A. The primary care sports medicine fellowship: American Medical Society for Sports Medicine proposed standards of excellence. British Journal of Sports Medicine. 2017;**51**(18):1328-1337. DOI: 10.1136/bjsports-2016-097428

[4] Thornton JS, Frémont P, Khan K, Poirier P, Fowles J, Wells GD, et al. Physical activity prescription. A critical opportunity to address a modifiable risk factor for the prevention and management of chronic disease: A position statement by the Canadian Academy of Sport and Exercise Medicine. Clinical Journal of Sport Medicine. 2016;**26**(4):259-265. DOI: 10.1097/JSM.0000000000000363

[5] Pigozzi F. Specialisation in sports medicine: The state of the Sport Medicine Specialty Training Core Curriculum in the European Union. British Journal of Sports Medicine. 2009;**43**(14):1085-1087. DOI: 10.1136/bjsm.2008.055350

[6] Orrow G, Kinmonth AL, Sanderson S, et al. Effectiveness of physical activity promotion based in primary care: Systematic review and metaanalysis of randomised controlled trials. BMJ. 2012;**344**:e1389. DOI: 10.1136/bmj.e1389 (Published 26 March 2012)

[7] Jaques R, Loosemore M. Sports and exercise medicine in undergraduate training. Lancet. 2012;**380**(9836):4-5. DOI: 10.1016/S0140-6736(12)60992-1

[8] Cullen M, Mcnally O, Neill SO, et al. Sport and exercise medicine in undergraduate medical schools in the United Kingdom and Ireland. British Journal of Sports Medicine. 2000;**34**(4):244-245. DOI: 10.1136/bjsm.34.4.244

[9] Pandya T, Marino K. Embedding sports and exercise medicine into the medical curriculum; a call for inclusion. BMC Medical Education. 2018;**18**(306). DOI: 10.1186/s12909-018-1422-9

[10] Buckler DGW. General practitioners' training for, interest in, and knowledge of sports medicine and its organisations. British Journal of Sports Medicine. 1999;**33**:360-363. DOI: 10.1136/bjsm.33.5.360

[11] Baby B. What is sports medicine? Medical students don't know. British Journal of Sports Medicine. 2000;**34**. DOI: 7. DOI: 10.1136/bjsm.34.1.73-a

[12] Hardt F. State of primary care sports and exercise medicine in Brazil. British Journal of Sports Medicine. July 2018;**52**(14). DOI: 10.1136/bjsports-2015-095826

[13] Dijkstra HP. The role of the specialist sports medicine physician in elite sport. Aspetar Sports Medicine Journal. February. 2014;**3**(1):24-31

[14] Lobelo F et al. Routine assessment and promotion of physical activity in healthcare settings. A scientific statement from the American Heart Association. Circulation. 2018;**137**(18):e495-e522. DOI: 10.1161/CIR.0000000000000559

[15] Macleod DAD. Intercollegiate board for sport and exercise medicine.

British Journal of Sports Medicine. 2000;**34**(4):235. DOI: 10.1136/bjsm.34.4.235

[16] Recommended Curriculum Guidelines for Family Medicine Residents Musculoskeletal and Sports Medicine. AAFP Reprint No. 265

[17] Finnoff JT, Hall MM, Adams E, et al. American Medical Society for Sports Medicine (AMSSM) position statement: Interventional musculoskeletal ultrasound in sports medicine. British Journal of Sports Medicine. 2015;**49**:151. DOI: 10.1136/bjsports-2014-094219

[18] Team Physician Definition, Qualifications, and Responsibilities: Consensus Statement. Statement, I. 2014. American Academy of Orthopedic Surgeons

[19] Pohl DJ et al. Olympic games: Special considerations—Medical care for Olympians. In: Rocha Piedade S, Imhoff A, Clatworthy M, Cohen M, Espregueira-Mendes J, editors. The Sports Medicine Physician. Springer, Cham; 2019. DOI: https://doi.org/10.1007/978-3-030-10433-7_45

[20] Sweden LA et al. The International Olympic Committee (IOC) consensus statement on periodic health evaluation of elite athletes. Clinical Journal of Sport Medicine. 2009;**19**(5):347-365. DOI: 10.1097/JSM.0b013e3181b7332c

[21] Shrier I. Strategic Assessment of Risk and Risk Tolerance (StARRT) framework for return-to-play decision-making. British Journal of Sports Medicine. 2015;**49**(20):1311-1315. DOI: 10.1136/bjsports-2014-094569

[22] Dijkstra HP, Pollock N, Chakraverty R, et al. Return to play in elite sport: A shared decision-making process. British Journal of Sports Medicine. 2017;**51**:419-420. DOI: 10.1136/bjsports-2016-096209

[23] Dijkstra HP, Pollock N, Chakraverty R, et al. Managing the health of the elite athlete: A new integrated performance health management and coaching model. British Journal of Sports Medicine. 2014;**48**:523-531. DOI: 10.1136/bjsports-2013-093222

[24] Budgett R. Healthcare challenges at an Olympic Games. British Journal of Sports Medicine. 2013;**47**:401. DOI: 10.1136/bjsports-2013-092364

[25] Budgett R. Emergency care at the Olympic Games. In: McDonagh D, Zideman D, editors. The IOC Manual of Emergency Sports Medicine. Chichester, UK: John Wiley & Sons, Ltd; 2015. DOI: 10.1002/9781118914717.ch1

[26] World Health Organization. WHO Global Recommendations on Physical Activity for Health. Geneva, Switzerland: World Health Organization; 2010

[27] Trost SG, Blair SN, Khan KM. Physical inactivity remains the greatest public health problem of the 21st century: Evidence, improved methods and solutions using the "7 investments that work" as a framework. British Journal of Sports Medicine. 2014;**48**:169-170. DOI: 10.1136/bjsports-2013-093372

[28] Pedersen BK, Saltin B. Exercise as medicine—Evidence for prescribing exercise as therapy in 26 different chronic diseases. Scandinavian Journal of Medicine & Science in Sports. 2015;**25**(suppl 3):1-72. DOI: 10.1111/sms.12581

[29] Sallis R. Developing healthcare systems to support exercise: Exercise as the fifth vital sign. British Journal of Sports Medicine. 2010;**45**:473-474. DOI: 10.1136/bjsm.2010.083469

[30] MacAuley D, Bauman A, Frémont P. Not a miraculous cure—Just good medicine. BMJ. 2015;**350**:h1416. DOI: 10.1136/bmj.h1416

[31] Hupin D, Roche F, Gremeaux V, et al. Even a low-dose of moderate-to vigorous physical activity reduces mortality by 22% in adults aged $60 years: A systematic review and meta-analysis. British Journal of Sports Medicine. 2015;**49**(19):1262-1267. DOI: 10.1136/bjsports-2014-094306

[32] Garrett S, Elley CR, Rose SB, et al. Are physical activity interventions in primary care and the community cost-effective? A systematic review of the evidence. The British Journal of General Practice. 2011;**61**:e125-e133. DOI: 10.3399/bjgp11X561249

[33] Anokye NK, Lord J, Fox-Rushby J. Is brief advice in primary care a costeffective way to promote physical activity? British Journal of Sports Medicine. 2014;**48**:202-206. DOI: 10.1136/bjsports-2013-092897

[34] Khan KM, Weiler R, Blair SN. Prescribing exercise in primary care. BMJ (Online). 2011;**343**(7828):10-11. DOI: 10.1136/bmj.d4141

[35] Jefferis BJ et al. Objectively measured physical activity, sedentary behaviour and all-cause mortality in older men: Does volume of activity matter more than pattern of accumulation? British Journal of Sports Medicine. 2008;**0**:1-8. DOI: 10.1136/bjsports-2017-098733

[36] Marcus BH, Ciccolo JT, Sciamanna CN. Using electronic/computer interventions to promote physical activity. British Journal of Sports Medicine. 2009;**43**:102-105. DOI: 10.1136/bjsm.2008.053744

[37] Elley CR, Kerse N, Arroll B, et al. Effectiveness of counselling patients on physical activity in general practice: Cluster randomised controlled trial. BMJ. 2003;**326**:793. DOI: 10.1136/bmj.326.7393.793

Chapter 3

Knee Dislocation: Comprehensive Rehabilitation Program after Two-Stage Ligament Reconstruction

Olga Łakomy, Robert Trybulski, Artur Gołaś and Aleksandra Żebrowska

Abstract

Knee dislocation is a multi-structure injury that usually requires surgical treatment. One of procedures is two-stage reconstruction that gives possibility to carry out rehabilitation after each of the stages in accordance with the requirements resulting from graft anatomy and biomechanics of the joint. The aim of the study is to analyze possibilities of using created rehabilitation program and to evaluate its effectiveness in a young woman who suffered an accident while practicing sports. The study of peak power shows differences between limbs primarily in maximum strength of the quadriceps muscle. With increasing load, differences in power in knee extension were 32, 17, and 61%. The rate of power development examination on force platform showed similar possibilities of operated and unoperated limb (best 19.5 cm test, 70–74 W/kg/s), however, in each subsequent trial operated limb achieved a worse result, which was not observed in healthy limb. Good results in Lysholm and IKDC 2000 knee assessment questionnaire (in sequence 95 and 81.6 points) 6 months after completed rehabilitation indicate good functional preparation of the joint, which is additionally confirmed by the jump test. Peak power test indicates the need to increase the elements of strength and endurance training in rehabilitation.

Keywords: knee dislocation, two-stage reconstruction, PCL, ACL, rehabilitation after reconstruction

1. Introduction

In light of epidemiological studies, 30% of joint injury cases concern knee joints. Of all knee ligament reconstructions, anterior cruciate ligament (ACL) reconstructions account for 80%, with 65% cases occurring during physical activity, both during recreational activity and practicing sports [1]. The most frequent injury mechanism is twisting movement at stabilized foot and flexed knee. Knee dislocation is usually connected with the impact of substantial external forces and is characterized by permanent or temporary losing the contact by the opposite articular surfaces [2]. In order for the injury to be categorized as dislocation, at least two of four ligaments that stabilize knee joint should be torn [3]. This injury is connected with the damage of various articular structures, sometimes also neurological and vascular.

Crucial ligaments protect the knee joint from excessive anterior-posterior translation. The posterior cruciate ligament (PCL) ensures the major force that resists the posterior drawer effect (95% of the force), whereas the anterior cruciate ligament (ACL) prevents the anterior drawer displacements and overextension of the leg in the knee joint [4]. The ligaments interweave with each other, thus limiting internal rotation of the knee. Another function of cruciate ligaments is also initiation of the correct sliding of the joint surfaces in the direction opposite to the rolling motion. Two collateral ligaments control joint displacements in the frontal plane: tibial collateral ligament, which prevents from the valgus movement, and fibular collateral ligament, preventing from the varus movement, with the most effective stabilization observed at the extended knee.

Structural deformation and the related functional failure of the ligament typically lead to the development of joint instability, termed disturbed joint movement control. In the case of tearing an individual ligament, the instability pattern is simple (e.g. tibial collateral ligament rupture: medial instability) or rotational (ACL rupture: anterior-medial-anterior-lateral instability). Knee dislocation with damage to all the stabilizing elements represents a complex instability: in addition to all the above types of instability, additional anterior-lateral-posterior-lateral instability and anterior-medial-posterior-medial instability are also observed [5].

Conservative therapies and surgical interventions have been used in the treatment of cruciate ligament injuries. The conservative treatment is used in the case of partial ligament damage, without substantial symptoms of joint instability in people with low physical activity aged over 40 years of age, leading little active lifestyles [6]. In the case of acute injuries, conservative treatment is aimed to eliminate edema, joint hydrarthrosis, and pain syndromes, ensuring proper and painless joint mobility and adequate muscular tension and neuromuscular control (proprioception).

The surgical interventions are used in patients with positive results of functional tests for evaluation of anterior cruciate ligament, such as the Lachman test, the anterior drawer test, and the pivot-shift test with coexistence of subjective symptoms of instability reported by patients during the interview, such as knee giving way. In young patients, especially those who are involved in sports, the sufficient indication for the surgery is ligament rupture diagnosed during a diagnostic examination using magnetic resonance (MR) or ultrasonography examinations.

An integral part of the patient treatment process is preoperative and postoperative rehabilitation. The procedures before the surgery are mainly aimed to obtain the range of joint motion needed for the reconstruction, prevent muscle atrophy, increase muscle strength, and improve proprioception. Early postoperative rehabilitation accelerates recovery and is usually started a day after the surgery. This procedure impacts significantly on reducing the time of patient's regaining full health [7, 8].

2. Study aim

In the case discussed in the study, patient's knee dislocation led to breaking the anterior and posterior cruciate ligament and fibular and tibial collateral ligaments with grade 1 injury to the medial meniscus (X-ray, MRI). For this complex injury, followed by multiple-stage treatment, an individual rehabilitation program was developed, with consideration for the type of injury, time between injury and the first and another reconstruction, method to perform reconstruction and available orthopedic aids. The aim of the study is to analyze the possibilities of using a comprehensive rehabilitation program and to evaluate its effectiveness after a two-stage reconstruction of knee ligaments.

3. Material and methods

The patient was female, aged 28 years, with body height of 170 cm and body mass of 55 kg (BMI 18.69). The injury occurred during a sport climbing activity due to the insufficiently protected landing surface. The training experience was 10 years of climbing, the trainings were usually completed three times a week with endurance components (running, swimming). Based on the information collected during the interview, the patient was a physically and professionally active person, which had a significant effect on the level of determination in activities leading to full recovery. The patient was qualified by the case physician for operative intervention. The entire process of diagnosis and surgical treatment was supervised by the same orthopedic surgeon and the surgery was performed in the same medical center.

3.1 Medical procedure and rehabilitation

After diagnostic examinations (knee joint X-ray examination) and excluding the damage of the popliteal artery and the peroneal nerve (ultrasound diagnosis of the popliteal fossa), the knee was reset into the proper position and immobilized by means of a knee joint immobilization bar (Sporlastic Genustabil 0°). A week later, the MRI examination revealed ruptured anterior cruciate ligament (ACL), posterior cruciate ligament (PCL), and fibular and tibial collateral ligaments (MCL) with grade 1 injury to the medial meniscus. The operating intervention involved two separate reconstruction procedures. The first one concerned the posterior cruciate ligament, whereas the second was used to reconstruct the anterior and fibular ligaments. An additional procedure used before the reconstruction was arthroscopy in order to remove arthrofibrosis.

The individual program of rehabilitation developed for the purposes of the discussed case took into consideration the damages to all structures formed during the injury, guidelines of the case physician, and the basic principles of rehabilitation [9]. The complete rehabilitation procedure was divided into four stages.

The first stage directly after the injury lasted 10 weeks. The most important elements of the rehabilitation procedure together with the marked moment of their implementation are presented below (**Table 1**).

Due to the damaged falciform cartilage, the first stage focused on creation of the conditions for the cartilage growth: immobilization of the joint for 4 weeks, complete absence of the load to the limb. At this stage, the activities also involved stimulation of creation of the scar in the location of the tibial collateral ligament through transverse massage (this ligament is fused with the joint capsule and the correctly formed scar can successfully overtake the function of the ligament). An additional recommendation in the period of immobilization was to use a Medi PTS orthosis, which ensured complete extension of the leg and, through the special pad fixed under the knee, it pushed the lower leg to the front, thus preventing the joint capsule contraction. Preparation of the joint for posterior cruciate ligament reconstruction was started after 4 weeks from immobilization and consisted mainly in reaching 100–110° of relaxed flexion movement in the knee joint (the range required for reconstruction). After around 2 weeks and reaching 90°, the meniscal block was observed. After consultation with the doctor, the meniscus was excluded as a cause of mobility limitation and, since the range of motion needed for the reconstruction was not achieved, the arthroscopy was performed to remove arthrofibrosis.

After the arthroscopy which was performed to remove the resulting arthrofibrosis (ROM 0–80), the second stage of rehabilitation was started for 6 weeks and focused on the preparation of the joint and limb for reconstruction (**Table 2**).

Stage 1: directly after the injury: MRI: total rupture of ACL, PCL, MLC, PLC, grade 1 injury to the medial meniscus.

Procedure	Time after injury (weeks)	1	2–4	5–7	8–10
PRICE and kinesiotaping (to reduce hematoma and edema)		+			
Elimination of the load to the joint		+	+		
Immobilization using Medi PTC (day/night) orthosis		+/+	+/+	−/+	−/+
Isometric exercises		+	+		
Stretching (to remove muscle tone) of muscles of rear and medial parts of the thigh		—	+	+	+
Joint mobilization (0–60°): passive, self-controlled exercises, patella mobilization		—	—	+	
Partial loading/learning to walk on crutches		—	—	+	
Proprioception learning		—	—	+	+
Full load		—	—	—	+
Further joint mobilization (>60°): active exercises in closed kinematic chain (CKC), mobilization		—	—	—	+

Table 1.
The first stage of rehabilitation.

Stage 2: following the arthroscopy aimed to remove arthrofibrosis and ACL stump debridement

Procedure	Time after injury (weeks)	Day 1–3	1–2	3+
PRICE and kinesiotaping (to reduce edema)		+		
Joint mobilization (>90°): passive, self-controlled exercises		+		
Partial loading		+	+	
Immobilization using Medi PTC (day/night) orthosis		−/+	−/+	−/+
Isometric exercises		+	+	
Stretching (to remove muscle tone) of the hamstring muscles		—	+	+
Proprioception learning		—	+	+
Full load		—	—	+
Strengthening exercises (load + CKC)		—	—	+

Orthosis Jack PCL worn over the day from the second week.

Table 2.
The second stage of rehabilitation.

The procedure following the arthroscopy was oriented at reaching 110° of the knee flexion as soon as possible. The active joint movement on the first day following the intervention was ca. 70°, which was a good prognosis for further improvement in mobility. The required range of motion was reached after 2 weeks. Therefore, active exercises were included, focused on increasing the strength of the quadriceps femoris muscles, hamstring muscles, and the gastrocnemius muscle. In order not to lead to tibia displacements with respect to the femur that are observed during muscle contraction, the exercises were performed only in closed kinematic chain (CKC). The elements of the proprioception training were also introduced (initially with partial load and then with full load), approaching it more as learning and preparation to the postreconstruction period. It was suggested that a dynamic orthosis (Jack PCL) that pushes the lower leg to the front with constant force during limb loading and knee movements should be used for the remaining 4 weeks after the surgery.

The third stage started just after the reconstruction of the posterior cruciate ligament. The components of the rehabilitation procedure together with the time interval in which they were introduced for therapy are presented in **Table 3**. Attention can be paid, among others, delayed mobilization and loading of the limb.

Four months after the injury, PCL was already reconstructed. For the first 2 weeks, the isometric contraction of the quadriceps femoris muscles, thigh adductors, and knee flexors was performed. The knee joint during these exercises was slightly flexed and a pad was inserted under the lower leg to push the tibia forward. Similar extension of the knee joint occurred at a light knee flexion. The iliotibial band was relaxed manually and the patella was mobilized. All these interventions were continued for the following weeks. After 2 weeks, the passive movement in the joint was introduced, with the range of 10–30°. This is the range of motion in which none of the parts of the anterior cruciate ligament are tensed. During passive movements in the open kinematic chain, the tissues of the anterolateral fascicle are contracted up to 30°, whereas for the posteromedial fascicle—at full extension [10]. In order to maintain knee extension, the exercises of extension in the range of 30–0° were performed in closed kinematic chain (pressing the foot against the mattress leaning against the wall; later, the mattress was replaced with a ball). Closing the system and pressing the articular surfaces against each other minimized tension of the posteromedial fascicle (safe range of motion for the posterior cruciate ligament in the closed chain is 0–60°, [11]). After 4 weeks, these exercises were performed in partial load to the limb (using the crutches/ladder). With the reduced graft strength [12], the patient was informed about the absolute prohibition of performing the twisting movement of the limb, waving the limb, and maintaining relaxed limb in the standing position. The patient was wearing the orthosis all the time (the orthosis was removed only for the time of exercises), initially using the Medi PTS and, when the hydrarthrosis reduced, Jack PCL was used over the night and Medi PTS was worn at night. Joint mobilization was started after 8 weeks. Although the threshold of 30° was not exceeded for a long time, the knee responded very well to passive movements, with the range of motion increasing gradually (it was 0–90 after 2 weeks). Furthermore, the patients performed exercises that supported flexion combined with active extensions at home, in the lying position, with the healthy leg resting on the wall at a right angle and the operated leg (straight) moved downward sliding on the wall and returning to the initial position (initially the healthy leg put under the heel of the operated leg). After introduction of gentle joint immobilization in week 13, the flexion reached 120°. The focus was on increasing strength, with much work in closed kinematic chains in the range of 0–60 (the highest shear forces were recorded for 85–105°) and open kinematic chain (extension)—initially in the range of 0–30 increasing gradually to 0–75° (shear forces were the highest for 75–90°) and in flexion (due to high shear forces, it is safe to introduce them 4 months after reconstruction) [13, 14]. Wherever the hamstring group was engaged, the tibia was additionally protected against the posterior translation (counterpressure) [10]. The components of proprioceptive training were added, with gradually increased difficulty (by e.g. more unstable ground, i.e. patient distraction) and the elements of preoperative patient's activity were added. From week 15, the patients exercised on her own, focusing on increasing the strength and muscle endurance. All the exercises except for proprioceptive training were performed while wearing a Jack PCL orthosis (at maximal lower leg pushing

Stage 3: following the PCL reconstruction (*double-strand ST and G tendons, TightRope fixation with bioabsorbable screw, tibia-interference screw (bioabsorbable), additional fixation: bone bridge with Hi-Fi suture thread, repair of posteromedial fascicle of the PCL using the titanium anchor with double Hi-Fi suture thread)*

Procedure	Time after injury (weeks)	Day 1–3	1–2	3–4	5–6	7–8	9–10	11–15	16+
PRICE and kinesiotaping (to reduce edema)		+							
Joint immobilization		+	+						
Isometric exercises of the quadriceps femoris muscle and adductors of the hip*,**		+	+						
Stretching exercises of the muscles of the hamstrings and the calf*,**		+	+	+	+	+			
mobilization of the patella and iliotibial band (ITB), prevention of the patellofemoral pain syndrome (PFPS)		—	+	+	+	+	+	+	
Passive exercises in the range of 10–30°		—	—	+	+	+			
Passive exercises of extension in CKC in the range of 0–30°**		—	—	+	+	+			
Partial loading		—	—	—	+	+			
Proprioception learning		—	—	—	+	+	+	+	+
Joint mobilization (>30°): passive, self-controlled exercises (with active extension)		—	—	—	—	—	+	+	
Full load		—	—	—	—	—	+	+	
Strengthening exercises (load + CKC 0–60°)		—	—	—	—	—	—	+	+
Endurance exercises for the limb		—	—	—	—	—	—	—	+
Muscle strength exercises in the open kinematic chain (OKC) in extension (initially 30–0, next 75–0) and flexion		—	—	—	—	—	—	—	+

Medi PTS orthosis for first 4 weeks (24 h), and next (from the moment when load was added) Jack PCL orthosis worn over the day and Medi PTS worn at night.
**Performed in light flexion.*
***With counterpressure at proximal section of the calf (orthosis pad, therapist hands).*

Table 3.
The third stage of rehabilitation.

force). A clear surgeon's recommendation was used to this type of orthosis during all activities for half a year following the reconstruction.

The second stage of recovery of the knee joint stabilizing structure, i.e. ACL reconstruction combined with fibular collateral ligament reconstruction was performed 18 weeks following the anterior cruciate ligament reconstruction and it was the starting point for the last—fourth stage of rehabilitation. The rehabilitation proceedings differed significantly from the rehabilitation protocols after the reconstruction of the anterior cruciate ligament itself. Therapeutic elements, also with time reference, are shown in **Table 4**.

Orthopedic surgeon's recommendation was to immobilize the joint for 6 weeks. The procedure for the first 2 weeks differed from the previous stage, in that the lower leg was not supported in the posterior part in lying supine, and the isometric contraction was accompanied by co-contraction of the hamstrings. After 2 weeks, minimal flexion movements were added (passively, with the help of the therapist, 0–20°), with

Stage 4: following the reconstruction of ACL and PLC ***(ACL: middle third of the quadriceps femoris aponeurosis with bone block of the patella; fixation: thigh—7 × 20 mm titanium interference screw, tibia: 9 × 25 mm titanium interference screw, PLC (modified Larson's method) double-strand ST tendon from the contralateral limb; fixation: thigh—TightRope, peroneum—bone bridge around the peroneum with Hi-Fi suture thread)***

Procedure	Time after injury (weeks)	Day 1–3	1–2	3–4	5–6	7–12	13–15	16+
PRICE and kinesiotaping (to reduce edema)		+						
Joint immobilization		+	+					
Isometric exercises of the quadriceps femoris muscle and adductors of the hip		+	+					
Stretching (to remove muscle tone) of the hamstring muscles		+	+	+	+	+		
Mobilization of the patella and iliotibial band (prevention of PFPF)		—	+	+	+	+	+	
Passive exercises in the range of 0–20°		—	—	+	+	+		
Isometric exercises with co-contraction at full extension and slight flexion		—	—	+				
Partial loading		—	—	+	+	+		
Proprioception learning		—	—	+	+	+	+	+
Joint mobilization >20°: passive, self-controlled exercises (with active extension)		—	—	—	+	+	+	
Full load		—	—	—	+	+	+	
Correct gait exercises, exercises for proprioception with load		—	—	—	—	+	+	
Active exercises in CKC in the range of 0–60° with co-contraction		—	—	—	—	+	+	+
Vigorous muscle strength exercises in CKC, 0–90		—	—	—	—	—	+	+
Muscle strength exercises in OKC in extension (without range 30–0) and flexion (20–90)		—	—	—	—	—	+	+
Endurance exercises for the limb		—	—	—	—	—	+	+

Medi PTS orthosis worn for first 2 weeks (24 h), without the pad pushing the lower leg forward, and next (from the moment when load was introduced) Jack PCL orthosis worn over the day (with minimal pushing force) and Medi PTS worn at night.

Table 4.
The fourth stage of rehabilitation.

the isometric contractions with co-contraction of the hamstring muscles performed in full extension and in flexion of ca. 15°. Light flexion also allowed for proprioception exercises without load. Early introduction of the components of proprioceptive training (preferably already in the acute phase) accelerates regaining muscular control, which, with the knee extension, minimizes the risk of patellofemoral pain syndrome, and allows for maintaining the proper gait pattern [15]. Joint mobilization was started in the week 6. The large part of time was devoted to the improved proprioception: initially more in the sitting position and lying supine using balls and next in standing on the unstable ground (sensorimotor pads, mattresses with various softness, or platform for balance exercises) with both feet and then standing on one leg. Gait exercises were started after reaching the range of motion of 70° (ca. 2 weeks after mobilization started). Similar to the procedure following the PCL reconstruction, the focus was on gait symmetry and balance elements were added. Exercises of muscle force in closed kinematic chains were performed in the range of 0–60° excluding co-contraction of the hamstring muscles (half-squats with body forward inclination). In the 12th week, range of motion was 120°. After 12th week, new ligaments showed greater mechanical resistance [16], which allowed for introduction of muscle strength exercises with greater intensity: squats with load, mini-squats on one leg, and exercises with a stair stepper. Range of motion for the exercises in closed kinematic chain was 0–90°. In the open kinematic chain, the flexion movements were initially performed at 20–60°, whereas extension was 90–70° (the range was increased to 90–30° after ca. 4 months). No extension exercises were used in the range of motion of 30–0°, which leads to excessive tension of the graft [17]. Endurance training was also introduced (stair stepper, cycle ergometer) and components of proprioception training were extended by the components of various sports.

3.2 Subjective assessment of the effects of rehabilitation (Lysholm i IKDC 2000 questionnaires)

The patient was asked to evaluate the functioning of the knee joint twice: immediately after the completion of the fourth stage of rehabilitation (study 1) and then after 18 months (study 2). Two scales were used for the assessment: the knee joint assessment scale according to Lysholm and the IKDC 2000 knee assessment questionnaire (The International Knee Documentation Committee 2000). Both contain information about knee joint ailments and their impact on the functioning of the patient in daily life.

3.2.1 Lysholm knee scoring scale

The Lysholm scale contains eight points concerning pain and activity. In each point, the examined person is supposed to choose and check one of the statements which matches his or her pain or functions, each answer is a specific number of points. Maximal total score is 100 points, which means the highest subjective functional status possible (perfect level–over 90 points). The following functional levels are good: 84–90 points, satisfactory: 65–83 points and insufficient: below 65 points) [18].

3.2.2 IKDC 2000 questionnaire

The IKDC 2000 subjective knee evaluation form is composed of three blocks, which concern: pain, physical activity, and function during activity of daily living (ADL). Similar to filling the Lysholm form, the patient is expected to choose and check one of the statements that matches his or her complaints and abilities. For each answer, a certain number of points is assigned according to the principle that

0 means the greatest ailments or the most limited function. Highest final score that can be achieved being also 100 points.

The questionnaires with the instructions concerning the method of scoring and interpretation of the result were collected from the website of the American Orthopedics Society for Sports Medicine [http://www.sportsmed.org/research/IKDC_forms/].

3.2.3 Evaluation of the peak power and rate of power development

The examinations were performed in the laboratory of the Academy of Physical Education in Katowice, 18 months following the last stage of rehabilitation. Peak power (P_{peak}) of the knee flexors and extensors of operated limb was evaluated and the results were compared with the measurement for the healthy limb. Keiser A-300 Leg Curl/Leg Extension system was used for the examination.

The methodology consisted in maximal flexion and extension in the position that allowed for examination of only knee joint movements, that is, isolated work of the hamstrings in the case of flexion and quadriceps femoris muscles (more specifically, vastus muscles, excluding the rectus femoris) in flexion. The second limb rested relaxed on the device and was not stabilized. The examination was preceded by a short warm-up and several repetitions of the movement without load. Healthy leg was examined first. After receiving detailed instruction, the patient was asked to repeat the test of maximal knee flexion at the load of 10 kg twice at 5 s intervals. Next, the test was repeated with the load increasing to 20–30 kg. The tests were repeated in order to evaluate strength of knee joint extensors using the same loads. One-minute recovery break was used before the tests.

Rate of power development was measured by means of the force platform Accu Power. The measurement was preceded with accurate measurement of body mass and body composition analysis. After stepping on the platform, the patient adopted the test position: standing on one leg (the healthy leg was examined first) and then, at the signal of the test supervisor, the patient jumped up. After landing, the patient left the platform and repeated the procedure twice in consecutive tests. Next, the examination was repeated for the other limb.

4. Results

The results of the questionnaires are presented in **Table 5**.

In the power tests, differences in peak power of quadriceps femoris muscle were found between the operated and nonoperated limbs. With the increasing load, the differences in power in knee extension were 32, 17, and 61% (**Table 6**). Examination of the power in the hamstrings also revealed smaller differences at lower levels of load between the legs. The use of maximal tolerable load of 30 kg confirmed greater difference in power at the level of 15% (**Table 6**). **Tables 6** and 7 include better result of the two attempts performed during the test.

Scale	Points	
	Test number 1	Test number 2
Lysholm	85	95
IKDC 2000	78.2	81.6

Table 5.
The results of the questionnaires.

Intensity	Power [W]		Differences %
	Right lower limb (following the reconstruction)	Left lower limb (healthy)	
10 kg	128	169	32
20 kg	196	231	17
30 kg	156	251	61

Table 6.
Quadriceps femoris power (knee extension).

Intensity	Power [W]		Differences %
	Right lower limb (following the reconstruction)	Left lower limb (healthy)	
10 kg	77	78	1
20 kg	139	148	6
30 kg	137	157	15

Table 7.
Hamstring power (knee flexion).

Analysis of the jump height using the right (operated) limb and the nonoperated limb revealed differences in rate of power development achieved in consecutive tests. The highest power was recorded for the operated limb during the first jump (19.5 cm; 70.6 W/s/kg), with power reducing for consecutive tests to 18.7 cm, (67.9 W/s/kg) and 16.3 cm (59 W/s/kg), respectively. During the examination of the healthy limb, the values obtained in the first and second tests were lower compared to the operated limb, with 16.5 (62.7 W/s/kg) and 17 cm (64 W/s/kg), respectively. The power similar to that of the operated limb was obtained only for the third attempt, with its value reaching 19.5 cm (74 W/s/kg).

5. Discussion

5.1 Methods of surgical treatment

Knee joint dislocations account for fewer than 0.2% of all orthopedic injuries [19]. Collecting a numerous group of participants which would be homogeneous in terms of treatment methods in order to perform a detailed analysis is extremely difficult. Most studies have analyzed small groups of patients, which prevent from finding the best treatment options for knee joint displacement [20].

The doubts during the choice of the treatment method concern mainly the timing and stages of the interventions. Most studies that have demonstrated the advantage of sutures or ligament reconstruction in the acute phase (first 2–3 weeks following the injury) have examined only the anterior cruciate ligament. In the case of dislocation, Liow et al. [21] compared ACL and PCL stability and range of motion of the knee joint between two groups of patients: one group with the intervention in the acute phase (up to 2 weeks following the injury) and the other with the reconstruction performed following at least 6 weeks. The authors documented improved ACL stability for the intervention in the acute phase (first 2 weeks) and no significant differences in PCL stability. No differences were also found in mobility between both groups. In light of general knee function, the levels of activity and anterior tibial translation, the results were better in the knees reconstructed within 2 weeks from the injury [21]. Another problem concerning the acute phase of the dislocation is the decision on suturing or reconstruction of the ligament. Sutures should be placed within 3 weeks following the injuries since scarring make the operation more difficult. It would seem that a torn ligament with preserved insertions can be more advantageous situation than a graft fixed in the bone tunnel. Furthermore, Mariani et al., in a study of 23 patients, demonstrated better outcomes in patients following total reconstruction of ACL and PCL compared to those after direct repair of the cruciate ligaments [22].

The attempt to perform a longitudinal analysis (12 years) of the results of treatment of knee joint dislocations and determination of prognostic factors for the results was started by Hirschmann et al. [23]. In a study of 68 patients, the researchers demonstrated a high effectiveness of the on-stage ligament reconstruction and indicated the correlation of the results with the demographic factors (e.g. age, education, and social status), body build (BMI), injury pattern (number of torn ligaments, damage to other structures), and operating timing. The factors that predispose to worse results include damaged fibular collateral ligament, combined reconstruction of ACL and PCL (according to the authors, most patients did not need PCL reconstruction), and delayed interventions > days [23]. Bin and Nam [11] presented very good results concerning the range of motion and stability in patients who underwent two-stage ligament reconstruction. The first stage involved reconstruction of medial and lateral ligament complexes within 2 weeks following the injury. The second stage, 3–6 month later, after regaining full range of motion, consisted in ACL reconstruction and/or PCL reconstruction if the substantial instability was found [11].

5.2 Rehabilitation proceedings

Fewer studies and, accordingly, fewer questions, were asked concerning postoperative procedures. The publications cited have discussed techniques of performing surgical interventions and final results concerning stability of ligaments and joint mobility. However, they failed to provide information about rehabilitation. Hirshmann et al. examined simultaneous reconstruction and emphasized the necessity of immediate mobilization in order to prevent arthrofibrosis. These authors recommended applying partial load to the orthosis with incomplete extension (10°) continued over 6 weeks. The limited passive and active movement was initiated immediately after the intervention, but the exercises of the first active flexion began following 6 weeks [23]. A very similar program was proposed by Robertson et al., who emphasized particular supervision and greater caution during knee mobilization following a complex reconstruction of several ligaments compared to that after isolated graft of a single ligament [19]. Ibrahim [24] encouraged to follow a more intensive rehabilitation program, recommending CPM movements in the rail within 0–30° and active knee flexion beginning as soon as 90° is reached. As emphasized by this author, this aggressive program, combined with early reconstruction of cruciate ligaments and repair of collateral ligaments, is highly effective in young and active patients [24].

The above examples suggest an overall idea of therapy following the complex reconstruction. However, there are no detailed protocols described after the interventions. It is known that some elements of therapy following ACL reconstruction differ extremely from those following PCL reconstruction. They suggest posterior support of the lower leg after PCL reconstruction, with different ranges of motion, which must not be accessed during the exercises due to the highest shear forces in the joint or the necessity to evoke constant co-contraction of the hamstrings during exercises after ACL reconstruction. It seems to be impossible to develop an ideal therapeutic procedure to ensure protection of both ligaments following the simultaneous reconstruction. Therefore, an optimum is attempted to be found. However, it often leads to delayed onset of complications, for example, those concerning patellofemoral pain syndrome. If the patient's lower limb following the PCL graft is not adequately supported at the posterior part, the joint capsule contracture may occur in this region. Gravity force that acts on the lower limb during lying (e.g. sleeping) or activity of the hamstrings in the sitting position is among the causes of shrinking of the structures in the dorsal part of the joint. If the joint capsule shrinks, the lower limb will give way toward the posterior drawer, whereas fresh PCL graft will be unable to adapt to the new function in adequate conditions. Consequently, the biomechanical joint conditions will be changed and, despite the graft, the patella and its ligaments should overtake the function of preventing from posterior displacement of the tibia. This will lead to the progressing arthrosis of the patellofemoral and femorotibial joints, while efficiency of the quadriceps femoris muscle will be reduced [13]. Two-stage reconstruction that our patient underwent revealed differences in therapies following PCL and ACL reconstructions. The rehabilitation procedure discussed in detail takes into account the origin and quality of the graft (evaluated by the operating surgeon) and the gradual process of ligamentation (three periods: necrosis, collagen types I and II synthesis followed by collagen type III synthesis in the ligament, which is most similar to the primary ligament [25] and the meniscus which was additionally injured. Due to its damage, the first stage focused on creation of the conditions for the cartilage growth. As noted by Hwang and Kwoh, the best solution is to use less invasive methods, whereas correct rehabilitation leads to the desired treatment effects [26]. In turn, long immobilization of the limb in the third stage of rehabilitation was dictated by the force of the graft—determined by the thickness of the collected tendon, it was assessed as poor. It was recommended to immobilize the limb for 8 weeks in order not to apply load to the graft, because graft tissues are weaker during the first period (6–8 weeks) following the reconstruction. Infarction is observed, with the replacement tissue degenerated and disorganized. It is after 8 weeks (week 8–12) when the graft is revitalized and its mechanical value is improving. Therefore, in order to create optimal conditions for graft acceptance, the balance should be found between graft protection from the excessive tension and the movement that is needed for rehabilitation of any joint (it prevents arthrofibrosis, improves blood supply, and nutrition of the graft). It was demonstrated that insignificant joint tension is favorable since it stimulates formation of new collagen and arranges its fibers along the loading force, thus improving mechanical properties of the new ligament [16]. A large part of each rehabilitation stage was exercises in a closed kinetic chain. The characteristic pattern of CKC exercises is reflexive co-contraction of knee-flexing muscles and the quadriceps femoris muscle, with minimization of the shift of the tibia. Furthermore, during these exercises, the increase in the flexion in the knee joint leads to the increased contraction of the quadriceps femoris and higher contact surface of the patellofemoral joint, with the force acting on bigger surface, thus leading to lower pain in the joint [14]. Another typical element of rehabilitation after ligament reconstruction is proprioceptive training. Tearing the ligaments, which have numerous mechanical receptors, leads to substantial disturbances in proprioception. Only after reconstruction, the ligaments regain the sense of joint position (kinaesthesia) over the rehabilitation process, thus restoring the reflexive muscle stabilization [27].

5.3 Methods of joint functioning assessment

In practice, the most often tools used to assess the knee after rehabilitation are: functional tests, examination of the range of movement in the joint, questionnaires or, less often due to the required equipment, joint stability tests on the arthrometer. In this case on the week 15 after the intervention, the following functional tests were performed: jumps on one leg over an obstacle (different directions), long jumps on one leg, climbing a step, and running with directional changes. Apart from the test results, the quality was also evaluated (joint control during the movement, maintaining joint axis at landing). The examination was mainly aimed to subjectively evaluate joint functioning and was not analyzed in percentage values. Eastlack et al. [28] presented similar activities as tests of functional evaluation. They used maneuverability test, with the patient running across a flat surface on the 6.3 m square envelope, shuttle run (running over a short section with rapid directional changes on the operated leg to the opposite direction), crossover running over the short distance, jumping on one leg and triple jump. The measure of the dysfunction depending on the test is time difference in performing the task or asymmetry of the distance of the jump compared to the other side [28, 29]. Previous activities at the same level of intensity can be restored at 85–90% efficiency, at good proprioception, coordination and muscle balance, and without hydrarthrosis and pain during and after the exercise [17].

An important condition is also return to the full range of motion. After completion of the therapy, the patient was able to make full extension and 150° flexion (examination of passive motion) in the knee joint. The attention was attracted to substantial differences in circumferences. Long immobilization at individual stages led to muscle atrophy, whereas performing isometric exercises is insufficient to prevent this phenomenon. In this specific case, immobilization resulted from the simultaneous injury to the meniscus and the necessity of protecting the graft (evaluated as poor). The solution to the problems of protection of the grafted ligament is artificial grafts. Bielecki et al. [30] described simultaneous reconstruction of only the side complex and revision of ACL using polyester grafts (LARS) that allowed for an early and intensive rehabilitation. Active joint mobilization was used on the first day, with full loading and exercises that strengthen muscles of lower limbs. This procedure offered very good short-term effects (full range of motion, stable knee joint, no differences in circumferences), whereas differences were observed between the imaging examination (tibia displacement during MRI and positive score in the Lachman test) and subjective patient evaluation using forms [30].

To monitor the results of treatment, special scales are commonly used to assess subjective complaints of patients. In the discussed case, the patient submitted the knee joint to subjective evaluation of functioning. Both on the IKDC scale and Lysholm scale, higher (better) results were obtained in the later evaluations. On the IKDC scale, in the section of activities of daily living, the patient indicated some limitations due to the inability of performing the complete squat (squat position) or sitting on the heels. These activities were improved with gradual increase in the range of motion. On the Lysholm scale, the deducted points concerned, among other things, the knee giving way–the patient claimed that she experienced such problems during practising sports. Better result in the second evaluation was probably obtained due to the substantial (but still not enough) rebuilding the muscles in the operated limb.

Half a year after completion of the rehabilitation, the significant muscle deficit continued to have an effect on the evaluation of the peak power. The method proposed in this work is peak power test and the jump test on the force platform. Both in the case of flexion and extension, the value of peak power of the examined muscles was greater for the left (nonoperated) limb. In the case of flexion, the difference was so small that it did not necessarily result from the injury and immobilization. In the case of extension, the power of the right limb muscles was significantly lower, accounting for 76% of the left lower limb power, whereas for the loads of 20 and 30 kg, this was 85 and 62%, respectively. The relatively good results for the load of 20 kg are likely to have resulted from the warm-up or increased patient motivation. However, overall tendency of the examination is the increasing disproportion between the value of peak power and the load: with the increasing load, the patient experienced more difficulty to achieve the result for the right leg similar to the left leg. The weakening of the quadriceps femoris muscle in the operated limb can be additionally confirmed by comparison of the first and second tests of the performed movement. Better result for the right and left limbs was achieved in the first test. Furthermore, the differences between the tests were substantially greater in the case of the operated leg. This means that the leg is not able to perform the extension movement twice with the same peak power, as it is the case with the left limb. Interestingly, the result of the jumping on the platform was better for the operated limb. This can be explained by the fact that, apart from the muscle strength, jumping ability is determined by such components as coordination and muscle balance, which may have resulted from the rehabilitation process which largely consisted in stabilization and working on the improved joint proprioception.

The proposed method of peak power test may turn out to be valuable information for both the physiotherapist and the patient himself. In the case of a significant deficit in the operated limb, it will be advisable to extend the therapy or individual work of the patient focused mainly on the muscle rebuilding. Then, the jump test seems to be a good tool for the functional assessment of the limb in players returning to the sporting activity.

6. Conclusions

Knee dislocation is quite a rare injury and therefore the choice of the treatment method raises many doubts. The choice of the method has an effect on the therapeutic treatment. The questions concerning the effectiveness of PCL reconstruction have been often raised among the authors of other studies due to frequent complications following the intervention. In our case, due to the age and athletic lifestyle of the patients, the necessity of restoring a complete stabilization apparatus seemed to be indisputable. A two-stage reconstruction allowed for different therapies following PCL and ACL reconstructions. Much attention was devoted to protecting of the PCL graft. The significant role in preventing complications was played by wearing an orthosis. The orthosis that pushed the lower limb forward (Jack PCL) following the injury and anterior cruciate ligament reconstruction seems to be necessary during therapeutic procedure: in certain private clinics, patients are refused to undergo the intervention until the orthosis is prepared. After completion of rehabilitation, the doctor evaluated the joint as stable in anterior-posterior direction (negative Lachman test, drawer test) with the first degree lateral instability. The patient was further recommended to gradually increase the load during training, care for maintaining muscle balance, perform exercises correctly, and continuously work to improve proprioception. The histological examinations demonstrated that the period of graft remodeling is 3 years and proprioception should be constantly stimulated in this period [16]. The power tests were expected to additionally evaluate the rehabilitation and point to the potential changes in the procedure (greater emphasis on strengthening of the limb following the periods of immobilization).

At the moment of the examinations, the subjective evaluation of the patient concerning joint functioning was positive, with the patient returning to full activity from the period before the accident. However, in order to fully confirm the positive final outcome of the used therapy, the examination with the evaluation of stability should be repeated after 5 and then after 10 years after rehabilitation is completed. It can be only stated that nowadays, the results of the tests with no pain symptoms and the lack of such symptoms during performance of the activities of daily living represent a good prognosis for a fast recovery.

Author details

Olga Łakomy[1], Robert Trybulski[2], Artur Gołaś[3] and Aleksandra Żebrowska[1*]

1 Department of Physiological and Medical Sciences, The Jerzy Kukuczka Academy of Physical Education, Katowice, Poland

2 Department of Medical Sciences, The Wojciech Korfanty School of Economics, Katowice, Poland

3 Department of Sport Training, The Jerzy Kukuczka Academy of Physical Education, Katowice, Poland

*Address all correspondence to: a.zebrowska@awf.katowice.pl

References

[1] Gianotti SM, Marshall SW, Hume PA, Bunt L. Incidence of anterior cruciate ligament injury and other knee ligament injuries, a national population-based study. Journal of Science and Medicine in Sport. 2009;**12**:622-627

[2] Bahr R, Krosshaug T. Understanding injury mechanisms: A key component of preventing injuries in sport. British Journal of Sports Medicine. 2005;**39**:324-329

[3] Brautigan B, Johnson DL. The epidemiology of knee dislocations. Clinics in Sports Medicine. 2000;**19**:387-397

[4] Czamara A. Functional benchmarking of rehabilitation outcomes following anterior cruciate ligament reconstruction. Ortopedia, Traumatologia, Rehabilitacja. 2010;**6**(in Polish, English abstract):519-533

[5] Lubowitz JH, Bernardini BJ. Current concepts review comprehensive physical examination for instability of the knee. The American Journal of Sports Medicine. 2008;**36**(Suppl 3):577-594

[6] Segawa H, Omori G, Koga Y. Long-term results of non-operative treatment of anterior cruciate ligament injury. The Knee. 2001;**8**(Suppl 1):5-11

[7] Dzierżanowski M, Hagner W, Biliński P. Proprioception as one of the factors determining the model of rehabilitation of patients after reconstruction of the anterior cruciate ligament. Ortopedia Traumatologia Rehabilitacja. 2003;**5**(Suppl 4):534-538 [in Polish, English abstract]

[8] Kruse LM, Gray B, Wright RW. Rehabilitation after anterior cruciate ligament reconstruction. A systematic review. Journal of Bone and Joint Surgery. 2012;**94**(Suppl 19):1737-1748

[9] Dale RB. Principles of rehabilitation. In: Andrews JR, Harrelson GL, Wilk KE, editors. Physical Rehabilitation of the Injured Athlete. Philadelphia: Saunders; 2012. pp. 41-66

[10] Milewska M, Mańka J. Proposal for a rehabilitation program after reconstruction of the posterior cruciate ligament of the knee using a simple thigh muscle tendon. Medicina Sportiva. 2002;**6**(Suppl 2):67-79 [in Polish, English abstract]

[11] Bin SI, Nam TS. Surgical outcome of 2-stage management of multiple knee ligament injuries after knee dislocation. Arthroscopy. 2007;**23**(Suppl 10): 1066-1072

[12] Ekdahl M, Wang JHC, Ronga M, Fu FH. Graft healing in anterior cruciate ligament reconstruction. Knee Surgery, Sports Traumatology, Arthroscopy. 2008;**16**(Suppl 10):935-947

[13] Fanelli GC. Posterior cruciate ligament rehabilitation: How slow should we go? Arthroscopy. 2008;**24**(Suppl 2):234-235

[14] Palmitier RA, An KN, Scott SG, Chao EYS. Kinetic chain exercise in knee rehabilitation. Sports Medicine. 1991;**11**(Suppl 6):402-413

[15] Timoney JM, Inman WS, Quesada PM. Return of normal gait patterns after anterior cruciate ligament reconstruction. The American Journal of Sports Medicine. 1993;**21**(Suppl 6): 887-889

[16] Woo SLY, Abramowitch SD, Kilger R. Biomechanics of knee ligaments: Injury, healing, and repair. Journal of Biomechanics. 2006;**39**(Suppl 1):1-20

[17] Kokmeyer D, Wahoff M, Mymern M. Suggestions from the field for return-to-sport rehabilitation

following anterior cruciate ligament reconstruction: Alpine skiing. The Journal of Orthopaedic and Sports Physical Therapy. 2012;**42**(Suppl 4): 313-325

[18] Paradowski PT, Roos EM. Scales of knee assessment. Basic concepts. Review of research methods. Linguistic and cultural adaptation. Ortopedia Traumatologia Rehabilitacja. 2004;**6**(4):393-405 [in Polish, English abstract]

[19] Robertson A, Nutton RW, Keating JF. Dislocation of the knee. The Bone & Joint Journal. 2006;**88-B** (Suppl 6):706-711

[20] Stayner LR. Historic perspectives of treatment algorithms in knee dislocation. Clinics in Sports Medicine. 2000;**19**(Suppl 3):399-413

[21] Liow RYL, McNicholas MJ, Keating JF, Nutton RW. Ligament repair and reconstruction in traumatic dislocation of the knee. The Bone & Joint Journal. 2003;**85-B**(Suppl 6): 845-851

[22] Mariani PP, Santoriello P, Iannone S, Condello V, Adriani E. Comparison of surgical treatments for knee dislocation. The American Journal of Knee Surgery. 1999;**12**(Suppl 4):214-221

[23] Hirschmann MT, Zimmermann N, Rychen T, Candrian C, Hudetz D, Lorez LG, et al. Clinical and radiological outcomes after management of traumatic knee dislocation by open single stage complete reconstruction/repair. BMC Musculoskeletal Disorders. 2010;**11**:102

[24] Ibrahim SAR, Ahmad FHF, Salah M. Surgical management of traumatic knee dislocation. Arthroscopy. 2008;**24**(Suppl 2):178-187

[25] Scheffler SU, Unterhauser FN, Weiler A. Graft remodeling and ligamentization after cruciate ligament reconstruction. Knee Surgery, Sports Traumatology, Arthroscopy. 2008;**16**(Suppl 9):834-842

[26] Hwang YG, Kwoh CK. The METEOR trial: No rush to repair a torn meniscus. Cleveland Clinic Journal of Medicine. 2014;**81**(Suppl 4):226-232

[27] Lephart SM, Pincivero DM, Giraido JL. The role of proprioception in the management and rehabilitation of athletic injuries. The American Journal of Sports Medicine. 1997;**25**(Suppl 1): 130-137

[28] Eastlack ME, Axe MJ, Snyder-Mackler L. Laxity, instability, and functional outcome after ACL injury: Copers versus noncopers. Medicine and Science in Sports and Exercise. 1999;**31**(suppl 2):210-215

[29] Rudolph KS, Axe MJ, Snyder-Mackler L. Dynamic stability after ACL injury: Who can hop? Knee Surgery, Sports Traumatology, Arthroscopy. 2000;**8**(Suppl 5):262-269

[30] Bielecki A, Płocki J, Pikuła D, Kotela I. Application of the LARS method to simultaneous reconstruction of the only-lateral complex and revision of the ACL of the knee joint—A case study. Polish Orthopedics and Traumatology. 2014;**79**:198-201 [in Polish, English abstract]

Section 2

Health and Exercise Medicine

Chapter 4

Interhemispheric Asymmetries and Individual Features of Regulatory Functions in Sport Psychology

Victor Moskvin, Nina Moskvina, Vladimir Nurgaleev, Zhanna Lukyanchikova, Vladimir Nepopalov, Elena Romanina and Vladimir Sopov

Abstract

In the chapter, the ontogenetic and psychophysiological features of the functions of volitional (arbitrary) regulation of behavior and its connections with the individual features of interhemispheric asymmetries are considered. Methodologically, the study of the peculiarities of human regulatory processes was based on the concept of partial domination of A.R. Luria and on the principles of neuropsychology of individual differences developed by Prof. E.D. Chomskoy and Prof. V.A. Moskvin who implemented the application of this approach in relation to sports activities. In this topic, over the past 5 years, we have conducted several separate studies of male subjects (mainly related to sports) of different age groups—adolescents, young men, and adult men (from 13 to 35 years old); the total sample size in general was more than 400 people. Methods aimed at identifying features of interhemispheric asymmetries (features of partial domination by A.R. Luria), psychophysiological and psychodiagnostic methods aimed at diagnosing individual characteristics (first of all, volitional qualities), and characteristics of arbitrary regulation, such as the R. Kettella test and others, were used. The research results revealed a predominant connection of regulatory processes with the structures of the left frontal lobe (in men) and the strengthening of this connection (increase in its significance) as the brain structures mature and mature.

Keywords: sports psychology, psychophysiology, brain, individual characteristics, functional asymmetries, young athletes, sports of the highest achievements, will, arbitrary regulation of behavior

1. Introduction

Will in psychology, as an independent mental phenomenon, is considered along with the mind and emotions. The problem of individual characteristics of volitional regulation is of great importance in psychology; it is also important in sports psychology in the selection and training of highly qualified athletes and has long been the focus of attention of sports psychologists [1–4].

However, it should be recognized that the problem of volitional regulation of human behavior still does not have an unambiguous interpretation both in general psychology in general and in sports psychology in particular.

In Russian psychology (in the Soviet period of development), the line of studying the volitional efforts of a person was successfully presented. Its representatives viewed effort as a central and specific sign of will. These studies began such scientists as A.F. Lazursky, M. Ya. Basov, further continued V.N. Myasishchev, V.S. Merlin in Russian psychology 50–80s of the twentieth century. It was also developed in the psychology of sports—A.C. Puni [5], P.A. Rudik [6], etc. trait of will. Despite the importance of these studies for their time, however, they can be considered obsolete due to the emergence of new areas of knowledge, such as neuropsychology [7, 8], as well as the neuropsychology of individual differences [9, 10]. Further studies have shown the possibility and prospects of applying this approach to the problem of arbitrary regulation in sports and sports psychology [3, 11–14]. This review presents the views of the leading representatives of Russian sports psychology on the problem of the will and new work in the field of differential sports psychophysiology regarding the possibility of studying the problem of volitional regulation of athletes taking into account the individual characteristics of hemispheric asymmetry [11].

2. Sport psychology about the problem of voluntary regulation

2.1 Avksentiy Caesarevich Pugni, Doctor of Psychology, Professor, representative of the Leningrad School of Sport Psychology (1898–1985)

A. Ts. Pugni singled out three components in the volitional act: cognitive (finding the right solution, self-assessment of the results of volitional actions); emotional (self-motivated, gain); and performing (physical regulation through conscious coercion) [5]. In the concept of Puni, the will is defined as "the active side of the mind and moral senses, allowing a person to control himself, especially in the conditions of overcoming obstacles of various degrees of difficulty." According to A. Puni, obstacles are a necessary condition for the actualization and development of the will. They arise as a result of the discrepancy between the capabilities of a person (his ideas, thoughts, feelings, and actions) objective conditions and characteristics of activity and are divided into external and internal. External obstacles were understood to mean any objective conditions and peculiarities of the external environment and activities that become an obstacle in achieving the goal, in solving particular problems; under internal obstacles—objective changes occurring under the influence of external conditions of human life and human activity and the state of the internal environment of his body, which serve as an obstacle to the achievement of goals. According to A. Puni, understanding of internal obstacles only as purely mental phenomena (adverse emotional and conflict mental states) is not always justified, since mental phenomena—secondary, derivatives, subjective side of objective changes, and the states of the internal environment of the body. External and internal obstacles interact, manifested in the difficulties of varying degrees [5].

2.2 Petr Antonovich Rudik, Doctor of Psychology, Professor, representative of the Moscow School of Sports Psychology, one of the initiators of the development of the psychology of sports in Russia (1893–1983)

He founded and headed the department of psychology at the GTSOLIFK (today the Russian State University of Physical Education, Sport, Youth, and Tourism), under his leadership, research was carried out in four main areas [6]. The first group includes studies of the characteristic features of various psychological processes, as essential components of physical exercises. The second includes experimental studies of some sensory processes and motor reactions in their relation to physical exercise. The third includes psychological studies on the problem of training exercise and sports training. And, the fourth includes research on the problem of education of the volitional qualities of the individual during exercise and sports.

P.A. Rudik considered will as the ability of a person to act in the direction of a goal, while overcoming external obstacles. In the minds of most people, the word "will" appears as a synonym for volitional regulation, that is, a person's ability to overcome difficulties that arise. About the will of man can be judged by how he is able to cope with difficulties. According to P. Rudik, will is the ability of a person to act to achieve a consciously set goal, while overcoming internal obstacles. Thus, the will is synonymous with volitional regulation, whose function is to overcome difficulties and obstacles [6].

Under the leadership of P.A. Rudik staff of the department of psychology, a number of scientific works on the problems of volitional regulation in physical education and sport were carried out. P.A. Rudik noted that studies of the problem of volitional training of athletes, conducted at the Department of Psychology, cover the following range of issues: (1) the psychological structure of voluntary actions; (2) the characteristic of volitional qualities of a person and the conditions of their formation; and (3) analysis of the process of education volitional qualities of an athlete.

In connection with these works in the 70s. the XX century Russian scientists have come to understand the fact that volitional training is part of psychological preparation, considered as a holistic reaction and as an integral part of the training process, does not cover the whole variety of mental functions. The incompleteness of this reaction in its scope, its attribution of teachers to the training process, the awareness of the need to take into account the various components of the psyche led to the separation of psychological preparation as a special education in the framework of training, and not the training process. It is within the framework of the preparation of the qualities required by an athlete that he can get his certainty; therefore, independence, acting as a training process, aimed at the formation of certain qualities, functions, and processes. Psychological training is carried out only by "improving" skills aimed at ensuring a certain state of fitness (or fitness). Training is always connected with the upbringing and development of moral and volitional qualities necessary for an athlete—willpower, will to victory, achievement of a goal, composure, perseverance, firmness in dealing with difficulties, decisiveness, courage, self-confidence, ability to manifest willpower, aimed at overcoming obstacles, discipline, etc. These volitional qualities are formed in the process of training, not as some abstract abilities but as related to the specific conditions of sports activity [6].

At present, due to the growth of professionalization of top-level sports and the revival of mass and youth sports, the study of the psychological basis for the development of strong-willed activity in sports, the basics of the process of strong-willed training of athletes in various sports taking into account their individuality and sports specialization research challenge.

The neuropsychological approach turned out to be more promising in this regard [7, 8], including taking into account the individual features of interhemispheric asymmetry [2].

2.3 Aleksandr Romanovich Luria, Doctor of Psychology, Professor, academician, one of the founders of the Faculty of Psychology and the Department of Neuro- and Pathopsychology of Moscow State University, as well as such areas as neuropsychology and cultural-historical psychology, a world-famous scientist (1902–1977)

His concept [7, 8] on partial domination of brain areas suggests that the basics of individual differences in healthy people are related to the variability of combinations of partial domination of sensory and motor signs (which determines their different contributions to the processes of realization of higher mental functions). To study the features of the functional asymmetries of man, AR methods are now widely used. Luria aimed at assessing "partial left-handedness" (or partial dominance of certain areas of the brain), as well as samples from other authors (for example, the modified Annette questionnaire) included in the "Map of lateral signs" [2]. The partial dominance of certain areas of the brain enhances the corresponding functions (including in the sphere of motor activity), which is also directly related to the problem of motor endowments in sports [2]. N. Sakano paid special attention to the sample of A.R. Luria "cross hands," which reflects the contralateral domination of the frontal brain [9]. And the frontal lobes are included in the third block of the brain, which is responsible for the functions of control, planning, and regulation of behavior [8].

Taking into account the features of functional asymmetries of the brain in sports activities is important in terms of identifying giftedness in certain spheres of the psyche (for example, in the motor sphere), which is associated with partial dominance of the frontal (motor) brain regions, especially its left frontal lobe. High-class athletes are educated at the level of limiting physical and mental stresses, which determines the deepening of the physiological mechanisms for improving the functional reserves of the human body in the process of adaptation to increasing loads and requires mandatory consideration of the individual characteristics of the athlete (including lateral ones) [2, 3].

The training of young athletes, taking into account their individual lateral profiles, is one of the central tasks of applying knowledge of neuropedagogics in sports [12]. Psychophysiological diagnostics of individual features (including motor ones) can be used to test and identify gifted children and adolescents in certain sports.

Human regulatory processes [8] to a greater extent associated with the third block of the brain, which includes the frontal divisions. Modern research confirms the existing opinion about the presence of asymmetry of brain blocks of Luria (including the third block). Today, it is established that regulatory aspects (at least in men) are mainly provided by the structures of the frontal regions of the left hemisphere. These provisions are confirmed by the data of psychodiagnostic studies of persons with different lateral features and the fact that the dominance of the left frontal lobe (in males) is associated with higher rates of formation of goal-forming functions [2]. Sample A.R. Luria is sometimes referred to as "Napoleon's test" by experts. It is interesting to note that Napoleon himself (who is considered to be left-handed) had, nevertheless, the right indicator of the "cross-hand" test, which, according to our data, implies a higher level of organizational and prognostic abilities and capabilities [2].

Today, at the Department of Psychology of the Russian State University of Physical Education, Sport, Youth, and Tourism, continuing the traditions of P.A. Rudik, further studies of volitional (regulatory processes) in athletes from the standpoint of the neuropsychology of individual differences [10] and modern sports psychophysiology [11–14] are being conducted.

New data were obtained that indicate the presence of individual features of communication and communication; a higher level of communicative abilities of athletes is mainly associated with left hemisphere dominance [14].

3. Research of human regulatory processes in sports

3.1 Individual features of the propensity to risk and impulsivity

Individual features of the propensity to risk and impulsivity were revealed by the example of students of a sports university [15] with different signs of dominance of the regulatory block of the brain according to A.R. Luria.

The experiment was attended by 80 students of the second year of a sports university at the age of 17–18 years old, of which 44 boys and 36 girls. The study of the individual psychological characteristics of the subjects was carried out using the following tests: questionnaire A.G. Shmelev (aimed at assessing risk appetite) and the questionnaire V.A. Losenkov, aimed at assessing impulsiveness. When analyzing the results of psychodiagnostic testing, the sample of students ($n = 80$) was divided into two subgroups with different indicators of the "cross of hands" sample—right ($n = 33$) and left ($n = 47$).

Analysis of the data showed that higher values of "impulsivity" were noted in the subgroup of subjects with left indicators compared with the right ones (49.38 and 46.97 points, respectively, $p < 0.05$) in the questionnaire of V. Losenkov.

The cognitive styles of "reflexivity-impulsiveness" were distinguished by J. Kagan in the study of intellectual activity, when, in the face of uncertainty, a decision had to be made and the right choice was needed from a number of alternatives. Impulsive people want to achieve quick success, which is why they tend to quickly respond to a problem situation. However, the hypotheses are put forward and accepted by them without careful thought; therefore, they are often incorrect. For reflexive people, on the contrary, slow response in such a situation is typical; the decision is made on the basis of carefully weighing all the pros and cons. Impulsive worse than reflexive, coping with tasks to solve problems, where no alternative answers are indicated. Reflexive are more independent than impulsive. They have a higher attention span. Impulsive have less self-control, low concentration of attention, but more volume. By willingness to take risks, one can understand the potential of the subject, manifested in the desire to act in situations of uncertainty, and it is successfully realized when it is possible to reduce this uncertainty through cognitive and personal efforts. Under impulsivity refers to actions and decisions taken on the first impulse, without first analyzing the situation (such decisions can also be called emotional). If we consider such personal property as a propensity to risk, then it can also be understood as a person's desire to choose situations of risk, danger, and uncertainty and to receive new and stronger impressions from it (associated with adrenaline rush). There is an analysis of the correlation between the concepts of "rationality" and "impulsivity." The trend of high rationality and low impulsivity, and vice versa, was revealed by prof. T. Kornilova both on the student sample and on the sample of teachers [15].

Many sports are associated with constant risk appetite. If we consider this concept more broadly, then it may reflect a common attitude to act in relation to various uncertain, risky situations. The readiness to resolve problem situations in the first place speaks of personal and social maturity.

3.1.1 Conclusion

According to the test data, it was found out that the right indicator in the "crosshair" sample correlates with lower "impulsivity" indicators for students at a sports university. This suggests the presence of individual differences in the features of the regulatory functions and indicators of impulsivity associated with inter-hemispheric asymmetries of a person. The results obtained can be used in the preparation of athletes, taking into account their individual characteristics.

3.2 Studies of the individual characteristics of control over the action associated with functional asymmetries

The features of control over the action [16] were studied on the example of students of a sports university (boys and girls 16–17 years old, n = 78) with different signs of asymmetry of the regulatory block of the brain according to A.R. Luria. For the diagnosis of volitional regulation, the "Kul's control scale" was used [17],which identified individual characteristics of control over the action, due to the asymmetries of the brain. The data obtained allow to conclude that lower emotional excitability, self-confidence (up to self-confidence), suppression of negative emotions, including the desire to avoid, move away, get out of situations that are extremely unpleasant and incompatible with human attitudes, to a greater extent associated with left hemispheric activation (right indicator of the sample "cross of hands").

The results are consistent with data from a study conducted by Y. Kul together with S.A. Shapkin and A.N. Gusev [17], who revealed left-hemispheric dominance of practically all components of self-regulation in the action-oriented subjects. When an unpleasant event occurs in the action-oriented subjects, the control system quickly identifies the unpleasant event, determines the degree of influence on the system (compared to other events), and alerts the mechanisms of the left hemisphere associated with the processes of preparation and control of motor programs. The authors believe that action-oriented subjects already at the early stages of processing stress information overcome the negative impact while maintaining a complex of relationships within the action control system (selective attention, emotional preferences, targeted representations, etc.).

The data obtained can be useful in the preparation of highly qualified athletes, (taking into account the individual characteristics of arbitrary regulation and control over the action in sports psychology).

3.3 Research of communication of volitional qualities and stability of motivation for playing football

Studied communication qualities and sustainability motivation to play football on the example of the 21st athlete-football (boys 15–16 years, n = 21). For the diagnosis was applied, the method "Color test" Luscher M., "Diagnostics of the motivational structure of personality" of Milman V., "Assessment of the relationship to the coach, the partners" of Marishchuk V.L. et al., "Analysis of the level of development of volitional qualities" of Puni A. Identified individual peculiarities of communication motivation to play football with the level of development volitional qualities of young footballers.

3.3.1 Conclusion

1. In football players aged 15–16 years old, the sustainability of sports motivation is promoted by:

    a. Pervasiveness and perseverance developed above the average, characterizing the stability of a motive as a motivational attitude and situationally manifesting stability of a motive, respectively, as well as endurance and self-control;

b. Attitude to the coach (except for the athletes of the group who are experiencing negativism, inadequate reactions, and resentment toward the coach);

c. The tendency toward frustration stability, predisposing to action in case of failures;

d. Willingness of the group for creative work (the motive of creative activity is the highest indicator of the motivational profile of a group of football players in general).

2. Reduce the sustainability of sports motivation:

a. Unproductive compensatory activity, tension, and frustration due to losing at competitions are compensated for by experiencing a negative attitude toward life and the demand to fulfill one's requests, otherwise the relationship is interrupted (except for the second subgroup);

b. The predominance of terminal motivation over procedural, including poorly developed motives of public utility;

c. Emotional passivity and multidirectionality within the emotional sphere (which is typical for young people), including associated with identified contradictions in motivational tendencies [striving for a high level of livelihoods with unwillingness to take active steps in the workplace (learning) activities].

The results can be used in the preparation of athletes, taking into account their individual characteristics and the level of development of volitional qualities of young football players [18].

3.4 Sports managers' goal-setting and psychological timing abilities

3.4.1 Background

Sport management may be described as the theory and practice of efficient corporate control in the sports sector, with the individual psychological qualities of a manager being crucial for the process success [19]. These qualities may include the following: time perception, timed prospects, goal-setting, field-dependence/independence, anticipation, etc. [2], and each of these qualities may be analyzed versus the individual interhemispheric asymmetries [2, 5, 6, 11].

3.4.2 Objective of the study

Objective of the study was to identify and rate the time perception variations in sport managers in the context of their individual functional asymmetries.

3.4.3 Methods and structure of the study

Subject to the study was a sample of right-handed highly educated mid-level sport managers aged 25–35 years (n = 30). The individual interhemispheric asymmetries were tested based on the Luria's Arms Folding Test [5], the test data being indicative of a domination of the relevant counter-lateral frontal lobe [2, 7]. Based on the Arms Folding Test Rates (AFTR), the sample was split up into the following two groups: Right AFTR Group and Left AFTR Group of 15 people each.

The time perception characteristics of the subjects were tested using the Time Semantic Differential Test (E.I. Golovakha and A.A. Kronik) [20] that implies the time perception process as the structure including the following three constituents: time continuity/discretion, time intensity, and the emotional attitude to a time range [20]. The study data were statistically processed using STADIA software.

3.4.4 Study results and discussion

The test data generated by the Temporal Semantics Differentiation Test showed notable differences only on the Time Intensity scale, with the Right and Left AFTR Groups rated by 19.4 points and 14.5 points on average, respectively ($p < 0.001$).

It should be noted that the time perception and timed prospects are known to be closely correlated with the goal-setting ability. As provided by A.N. Leontiev, a goal plays a system-forming role when an activity is designed, as follows: "Goal-setting process provides a key impetus for one or another subject activity"; with the goal-setting (goal-constructing) notion being defined as the "subjective identification of the goal that means the nearest target outcome for the subject activity that drives it forward" [19]. Such notion as anticipation (meaning the ability to foresee/predict a sequence of events) also plays an important role in the time perception, with the anticipation development level being generally considered indicative of the manager's mental qualities on the whole.

The above findings were supported by the relevant intellectual test data including the Raven's Progressive Matrices (RPM, a nonverbal group test) and Cattell's Questionnaire data. The test results may be explained by the higher level dynamic characteristics of the thinking process in the male subjects tested with the Right AFTR by the Hands Crossing Test [2]. We believe that the finding gives us reasons to state that the male subjects tested with the Right AFTR by the Arms Folding Test are more rational, self-reliant, and independent, plus more stable in the behavioral models they opt for. The individuals tested with the Left AFTR by the Arms Folding Test showed lower rates on a few test scales, the rates being indicative of the higher emotionality, egocentrism, field-dependence, sensitivity to stresses, and lower stability of the chosen behavioral models. The study data and analyses also showed their higher developmental rates in verbal intelligence, emotional stability, domination, self-control, field-independence, anticipation ability, overall internality, and self-management ability (including the goal-setting ability).

Our study findings may be interpreted as indicative of the sport managers with dominating left frontal lobe being more inclined to perceive and rate time in a more intense manner and, hence, expected to show higher self-management, self-control, and anticipation rates, i.e., the qualities of high professional value for a sport manager.

3.4.5 Conclusion

The study data may be applied for the differentiation diagnostics in the human resource screening/selection process for the sport management positions and for the vocational orientation purposes.

3.5 Study of individual peculiarities of regulation in young sportsmen of different ages

One of our last studies concerned the study of the individual characteristics of arbitrary regulation on the example of students of a sports university, taking into account the signs of functional asymmetries. Individual differences were studied in young athletes with regard to partial asymmetries according to A.R. Luria. To identify the individual psychological characteristics, a study was conducted with the help of R. Cettel's personal questionnaire (HSPQ); 45 teenagers 14–16 years old engaged in wrestling participated in the experiment. Of these, 25 subjects were with right-hand indicators of the "crossing hands" test according to A.R. Luria, which reflects the dominance of the left frontal divisions and 20 adolescents were with the left indicators of this test. The technique was also carried out on 110 students of 1–4 courses of a sports university at the age of 18–25 years (young men) also with different signs of asymmetry. It was revealed that the partial dominance of the left frontal lobe (both in adolescents and young men) is associated with higher indices of individual characteristics associated with volitional regulation.

3.5.1 Methods of research

The experiment was conducted in the form of group testing of two samples of subjects. To identify the individual psychological characteristics, a study was conducted using the personal questionnaire R. Kettell (adolescent version—HSPQ) in which 45 adolescents 14–16 years old engaged in wrestling participated. Of these, 25 subjects were with right-hand indicators of the "crossing hands" test according to A.R. Luria [7], which reflects the dominance of the left frontal regions (related to the arbitrary regulation of behavior) and 20 adolescents were with the left indicators of this sample. The study was conducted on the basis of the sports school of the Department of Physical Culture and Sports of Moscow [21].

A similar study was also conducted on 110 students of 1–4 courses of a sports university at the age of 18–25 years. For the study, the personal questionnaire was used by R. Kettel (Form A) and the indicators of the "cross-hand" test according to A.R. Luria. Thus, the total volume of the samples studied was 155 subjects. Statistical data processing was performed using the U-Wilcoxon-Mann-Whitney test.

3.5.2 The results of the study of teenage athletes

Comparison of the averaged data of the personal questionnaire R. Kettell (adolescent version—HSPQ) showed the following. According to factor E ("subordination—dominance"), higher values were noted in the group of adolescents with the right indicator of the "crossing of arms" sample—6.8 stan, in the group with the left indicator—5.2 ($p < 0.05$), which indicates about greater activity and leadership qualities of the subjects with the right indicators. The values for factor Q2 ("degree of group dependence") are higher in the group with the right symptom—6.6 stan, in the group with the left—4.3 ($p < 0.03$). The values for factor Q3 ("degree of self-control") are higher in the group with the right symptom—6.2 stan, in the group with the left—4.4 ($p < 0.03$).

3.5.3 The results of the study of students of sports universities

On the factors of the questionnaire R. Cattell (form A) were obtained the following results. According to the factor F ("expressiveness-restraint"), higher values were noted in the group of persons with the right indicator of the "crossing of arms" sample—5.5 stan, in the group with left—4.7 stan ($p < 0.03$), which indicates about greater activity, liveliness, and flexibility of behavior of subjects with the right indicator of the sample "cross arms". The values for the N factor ("naivety—insight") were lower in the group of people with right-hand indicators of the "crossing hands" test—5.1 stan, while in the group with left ones they were higher—5.9 stan ($p < 0.03$).

3.5.4 Discussion

In general, according to the results of the study, subjects with left hemispheric dominance reveal higher data on the R. Kettell method scales, which are associated with activity and self-organization, which in general may indicate a greater severity of indices of arbitrary regulation in this group of individuals.

The obtained data correlate well with the results of previously conducted psychodiagnostic studies. According to the data of the conducted experiments, it can be stated that as they mature (as they move from adolescent to older age groups), there is an increase in the indices of volitional qualities of the personality (in the method of M. Chumakov) and the indicators of the sustainability of the choice of color incentives. This is especially clearly manifested in the "left hemisphere" subjects (i.e., with the right-hand indicators of the "crossing hands" test) [2].

3.5.5 Conclusion

The obtained data can be successfully used in solving differential diagnostic problems in sports psychology, including the diagnosis of individual features of the regulatory functions of athletes.

The results show the presence of asymmetry of the third (regulatory) block of the brain according to A.R. Luria. This position is also confirmed by the data of psychodiagnostic studies of adolescents and young men with different lateral features [13, 21] and previously established data that the partial dominance of the left frontal lobe (often in males) is associated with higher rates of goal formation and volitional regulation. Our pilotage studies conducted earlier show that these indicators are less specific (more "blurred") for girls and women, i.e., they are not always confirmed by statistical processing. The results can be used practically to diagnose the individual characteristics of arbitrary regulation in sports psychology when training highly qualified athletes and to predict human behavior in extreme sports [2, 3].

3.6 Study of voluntary regulation and motivation achievement of success in young figures

Motivation to play sports is associated with many mental qualities, including their volitional characteristics [22]. Earlier, we noted that, according to psychodiagnostic studies, males with left hemispheric domination can identify higher levels of voluntary regulation, organization, risk appetite, focus on success, and higher levels of anticipation (or anticipation of future events) [2]. In sports psychology, such quality as the ability to anticipate and predict the development of future events is considered an important personal characteristic. Taking into account all the above, we conducted a study to identify the links of regulatory functions with the motivation to achieve success and other personal characteristics among teenagers-skaters (singles).

3.6.1 Research methods

The method of diagnostics of signs of partial domination according to A.R. Luria [7] was used (as a method of psychophysiological and neuropsychological diagnosis of the individual characteristics of human inter-hemispheric asymmetry). When implementing the method of psychological testing, we used the test of T. Ehlers (for studying the features of success motivation), the adolescent version of the test by G. Eysenck and the adolescent version of the R. Cattell method (HSPQ—for the study of the individual psychological characteristics of figure skaters). Statistical data processing was performed using the U-Wilcoxon-Mann-Whitney test.

3.6.2 The subjects

The study involved lone skaters aged 13–14 years (adolescent boys, n = 45). The subjects were divided into two subgroups: the first included subjects with a left hand cross-over indicator (n = 23), which reflects the partial dominance of the right frontal lobe related to the regulative block of the brain according to A. Luria. The second group consisted of subjects with a right-hand indicator of the "crossing of arms" sample according to A.R. Luria, which reflects the partial dominance of the left frontal lobe (n = 22). All subjects had approximately the same age and social status. The study was performed on the basis of schools of figure skating in the city of Vienna (Austria) [22].

3.6.3 The hypothesis of the study

Adolescent boys of 13–14 years old with right-hand indicators of the "cross-hand" test (which reflects the partial dominance of the left frontal lobe of the regulatory block of the brain) may show a higher level of motivation for success compared with adolescents with left-hand indicators of this test.

3.6.4 Purpose of the study

To study the features of the motivation to achieve success with single skaters (adolescent boys aged 13–14 years), taking into account individual psychological characteristics and profiles of functional asymmetries.

3.6.5 Results and discussion

3.6.5.1 Test T. Elers

In the aggregate of the characteristics of an effective sports activity, an important factor is the motivation to succeed. A real athlete with a high level of motivation is always at the center of any sports situation, and effective activity in any field implies a high degree of motivation.

The study of patterns and characteristics of the motivational sphere makes it possible to predict the behavior of an individual in a given situation. Therefore, the motivational sphere is one of the most important components of personality; it becomes the main object of study for psychological science in general and in the study of behavioral psychology in sports in particular.

According to T. Ehlers, the motivation to achieve success may manifest itself as follows: a person with a higher motivation to success prefers a medium or low level of risk, and he avoids a high level of risk. With strong motivation, the expectation of success is usually higher than with weak motivation; in their activities, people with strong motivation put more effort and energy to succeed, they show a desire for success.

On the scales of the T. Elers questionnaire, the following statistically significant differences were obtained (in terms of averages). In the course of the study, differences were found in the degree of manifestation of the level of motivation for achieving success in the "right hemisphere" ($n = 23$) and "left hemispheric" ($n = 22$) subjects, who were 15.2 points and 18.6 points, respectively, the differences are significant ($p < 0.05$). Thus, the indicators of motivation of the first group correspond to the average level of motivation to achieve success (for the "right-hemisphere," $n = 23$) and a higher level of motivation for achieving success for the second group of figure skaters (for the "left-hemisphere", $n = 22$).

3.6.5.2 Test Eysenck (adolescent version)

In the "right-hemisphere" skaters on the scale of "neuroticism-mental stability," this figure was 17.2 points, which corresponds to an increased level of neuroticism and indicates their higher emotionality. In the "left hemispheric" group, this indicator was 9.5 points, which corresponds to the normative indicators ($p < 0.05$). Differences in other scales between groups in this method were not identified.

3.6.5.3 The teenage version of the test R. Cattell (HSPQ)

For HSPQ factors, data were obtained: the "left hemispheric" skaters (as opposed to the "right-hemispheric") showed a higher level of emotional stability (factor C, 4.4 and 6.3 stan, respectively, $p < 0.05$); these adolescents are more self-sufficient and less dependent on the group (factor Q2, 4.5 and 7.6 stan, respectively, $p < 0.05$); they also show a higher level of self-control or volitional qualities (factor Q3, 5.3 and 7.2 stan, respectively, $p < 0.05$).

Thus, after analyzing the data obtained, the following conclusions can be made: the indicators of motivation of the "right-hemisphere" group correspond to the average level of motivation for achieving success and a higher level of motivation for achieving group success ("left-hemisphere" adolescents, $n = 22$). Psychodiagnostic indicators of "right-hemispheric" skaters ($n = 23$) show higher neuroticism indicators in Eysenck's technique, which indicates their greater emotionality and lower level of neuropsychic stability, which indicates a lower resistance to stress. The "left hemisphere" skaters ($n = 22$) have a higher level of emotional stability (factor C in the HSPQ test); these adolescents are more self-sufficient and less dependent on the group (factor Q2); they also show a higher level of self-control (factor Q3 of the HSPQ test), which indicates a higher level of development of volitional regulation, in contrast to the "right-hemispheric" skaters (the identified differences are significant).

3.6.6 Conclusion

The indicators of the "right-hemispheric" and "left-hemispheric" teenage skaters have significant differences related to the individual characteristics of inter-hemispheric asymmetries. In adolescent athletes with dominance of the left hemisphere, links were found between hemispheric dominance and a tendency toward authoritarian behavior, the presence of a high level of motivation for success, a tendency to take risks and to rivalry, a higher level of organizational skills. In the activity of right-wing athletes, organizational skills are less pronounced, they are more focused on avoiding failures than on achieving success. It should also be noted that these features (the connection between a higher level of arbitrary regulation and the motivation to succeed) are more clearly expressed in males; in women, these connections are not always so straightforward.

Thus, the hypothesis of the study that the motivational and volitional sphere of adolescent athletes is associated with the psycho-physiological features (individual hemispheric asymmetry) is fully confirmed; the goal of the study is achieved.

3.7 Regulatory functions and Internet dependence persons for student higher education

The problem of the regulation of the psyche is one of the main in modern psychology [2]. Deregulation is considered dependent forms of behavior (so-called addiction). Such manifestations as accentuation and psychopathization of a person in an unstable type are a pronounced manifestation of dependence and lack of independence. In clinical psychology, addictive behaviors are more studied on the example of chemical addicts (chronic alcoholism and drug addiction). Modern studies indicate a significant accumulation of signs of right-hemispheric partial domination of chemical addicts [2].

Recently, papers have emerged concerning the study of the characteristics of inter-hemispheric asymmetries in young Internet addicts. Analysis of behavioral reactions in groups of Internet addicts showed that dependent behavior is more typical of right hemisphere subjects and ambidexters. For groups with the right hemisphere specialization, the various parameters of addictive realization manifest themselves with a pronounced desire to violate the norms and social rules. Similar data were obtained in our study [2].

The literature data show that the features of functional asymmetries and the individual characteristics of psychological time in Internet addicts are still little studied. To study the individual characteristics of psychological time in this category of persons, we conducted a study with students of a sports university.

3.7.1 Hypothesis

A higher level of Internet addiction is associated with the predominance of right hemisphere dominance, which also affects the specifics of temporal perception.

3.7.2 The technique

To identify the possible connection of Internet addiction with the peculiarities of psychological time in a sample of young subjects (students of a sports university 18–17 years old, n = 100), the following psychodiagnostic methods were used:

1. Features of individual profiles of laterality, taking into account signs of partial dominance according to A.R. Luria (test "Map of lateral signs") [2].

2. The severity of Internet addiction (Kulakov S. test, 2004).

3. Features of time perception using the Zimbardo test (taking into account the availability of data on the individual features of the perception of time with different variants of the dominance of the right or left hemispheres) [2].

4. Individually psychological features using the test R. Cattell (form A).

(Other psychodiagnostic methods were used; however, these results are not considered in this article.)

3.7.3 Sample

Students from the 1–2 courses of the Russian State University of Physical Culture, Sports, Youth, and Tourism of 17–18 years old acted as subjects; the sample size was 100 people.

3.7.4 The results of the study

Currently, the study is ongoing, the data obtained are preliminary. As a result of the use of factor analysis, nine factors were identified (factorization completeness was 90%).

The factor "Behavior normativity" suggests that students with a predominance of right laterality (left hemisphere) in the motor and analyzer fields tend to behave in accordance with generally accepted standards, are able to foresee the possible consequences of their actions, are motivated to achieve future goals, and are ready to sacrifice today's pleasures for the sake of future success are more disciplined. High rates were noted on the "Normativity of Behavior" scale (factor G) of the R. Kettell test and on the "Future" scale in the F. Zimbardo's "Time perspective" method.

On the contrary, subjects with a predominance of left laterality (right hemisphere) in the motor and analyzing spheres are subject to emotions, disagree with generally accepted moral norms and standards, ignore duties, can act antisocial, inconstant, changeable, careless, lazy, independent, subject to influence unprincipled, irresponsible, and unorganized. Indicators of time perception are more related to the orientation to the present and the past.

3.7.5 Discussion

The data obtained are generally consistent with the proposed hypothesis. Earlier in our works, manifestations of left hemispheric insufficiency in individuals with addictive behaviors have been identified, which explains the weakness of predictive and regulatory functions [2].

We found that patients with chronic alcoholism tend to rate time as more discrete, less stressful, and less pleasant (compared to healthy subjects). The temporal orientation of patients is characterized by a lesser connection with the present and a greater orientation toward the past. In patients with chronic alcoholism, an abnormal distribution of individual lateral profiles is also detected. The results of our study of drug addicts show that there are significant differences in the nature of temporal orientations between drug addicts and healthy subjects. Drug addicts are more centered on the past and the present; the future is less significant for them. At the same time, drug addicted individuals feel time as less stressful (stretched, slowly flowing, empty, and unorganized) and less emotionally pleasant compared to healthy subjects. Assessment of drug addiction time is less pleasant due to the greater connection of the right hemisphere with negative emotions. The predominance of right-hemispheric functions in drug addicts can be explained by experiencing time as less stressful, since the left hemisphere is associated with a higher level of activity, and the right hemisphere is associated with relaxation and relaxation. It has been established that left-hemispheric individuals are more inclined to underestimate and re-measure durations compared to right-hemispheric individuals who are more inclined to overestimate and under-measure time intervals [2].

S.L. Rubinstein wrote that one of the most important components of the structure of personality is its focus [23]. The amorphousness and vagueness of life goals and the absence of a specific orientation of the individual can be considered as the soil on which different states of dependence develop. It is noted that the lack of volitional regulation and autonomy most often affects persons with an accentuation of the person of an unstable type who easily fall under someone else's negative influence, often drop out of school or work, alcoholize, or use drugs.

3.7.6 Conclusion

The research data testify to the weakness of regulatory processes in groups of Internet addicts and the accumulation of signs of right-brain partial domination in their sample. Thus, previously obtained data on the accumulation of signs of right-hemispheric domination in chemical addicts (in young people with manifestations of chronic alcoholism or drug addiction) [2, 24] can be extended to intensity addicts, which indicates the weakness of the functions of arbitrary regulation in them and says about the features of time perception in this sample. The stated results are preliminary (the main body of data is in the final stages of processing); however, they already indicate the presence of individual features of time perception in Internet addicts of a young age and can be used for differential diagnosis [25].

4. Conclusion

The obtained data allowed testing the methods of psychological and psychophysiological diagnosis of regulatory processes in sports. The research results confirm the prospects and productivity of the study of the problem of volitional regulation of athletes, taking into account the individual characteristics of interhemispheric asymmetry from the standpoint of differential sports psychophysiology [11].

The data show the presence of asymmetry of the third (regulatory) block of the brain according to A.R. Luria. This position is confirmed by the data of psychodiagnostic studies of adolescents and young men with different lateral features and coincides with previously established data that the partial dominance of the left frontal lobe (more often in males) is associated with higher rates of goal formation and volitional regulation. In general, the results of the research allowed to identify the preferential relationship of regulatory processes with the structures of the left frontal lobe (in men) and the strengthening of this connection (growth) as the brain structures mature and mature.

The presence of weakness in arbitrary functions of right-hemispheric Internet addicts also indirectly confirms the greater involvement of the left hemisphere in the arbitrary regulation of behavior (mainly in males).

The problem of individual features of voluntary regulation in female subjects remains unresolved, which may be associated with such a concept as "gestational dominant" (which provides the function of procreation), and which may have variable hemispheric localization. This requires further more in-depth research in this area.

Acknowledgements

The reported study was funded by RFBR (Russian Foundation for Basic Research), projects number 16-06-50146-a (f) and number 18-013-00856-a.

Conflict of interest

The authors have no conflicts of interest to disclose.

Author details

Victor Moskvin*, Nina Moskvina, Vladimir Nurgaleev, Zhanna Lukyanchikova, Vladimir Nepopalov, Elena Romanina and Vladimir Sopov
Department of Psychology, Russian State University of Physical Culture, Sport, Youth and Tourism, Moscow, Russia

*Address all correspondence to: 1700018v@mail.ru

References

[1] Rodionov AV, editor. Psychology of Physical Culture and Sports. Moscow: Academy; 2010 (in Russian) ISBN 978-5-7695-6833-6

[2] Moskvin VA, Moskvina NV. Interhemispheric Asymmetries and Individual Differences of a Person. Moscow: Smisl; 2011 (in Russian) ISBN 978-5-89357-303-9

[3] Moskvin VA, Moskvina NV. The problem of strong-willed regulation of athletes in the course of preparation of sports psychologists. Materials of the International Scientific-Practical Conference for the Workers of Science and Education «Education and Science-2016». Part 3. St. Louis, Missouri, USA: Science and Innovation Center Publishing House, 2016. p . 9-12. DOI: 10.18411/d-2016-047

[4] Sopov VF. Theory and Methods of Psychological Preparation in Modern Sports. Moscow: Department of Physical Education and Sport Moscow city; 2010 (in Russian)

[5] Puni AC. Psychological Basis of Volitional Training in Sports. Leningrad: GDOIFK; 1977. (in rus.)

[6] Rudik PA. Psychological Foundations of Moral and Volitional Training of an Athlete. Problems of Sports Psychology. Moscow: FiS; 1962. (in Russian)

[7] Luria AR. Higher Human Cortical Functions and their Disorders in Local Brain Lesions. 3rd ed. Moscow: Academic Project; 2000. 512 p. (in Russian) ISBN 5-8291-0079-7

[8] Luria AR. Basics of Neuropsychology. 5rd ed. Moscow: Academy; 2006. (in Russian) ISBN 5-7695-3073-1

[9] Sakano N. Latent Left-Handedness. Its Relation to Hemispheric and Psychological Functions. Jena: Gustav Fischer Verlag; 1982. 122 p

[10] Khomskaya ED, Efimova IV, Budyka EV, Enikolopova EV. Neuropsychology of Individual Differences. Moscow: Russian Pedagogical Agency; 1997. 284 p. (in Russian) ISBN: 5-86825-033-8

[11] Moskvin VA, Moskvina NV. Sports psychophysiology as a new direction of psychology. Sport Psychologist. 2015;**4**(39):10-14 (in Russian)

[12] Moskvin VA, Moskvina NV. Hemispheric asymmetry and principles of differential neuropedagogy in higher education. Materials of the International Scientific-Practical Conference for the Workers of Science and Education «Education & Science – 2016». Part 4 St. Louis, Missouri, USA: Science and Innovation Center Publishing House, 2016. p. 259-262. DOI: 10.18411/d-2016-048

[13] Moskvin VA, Moskvina NV. Psychophysiology and features volitional regulation sport university students. European Journal of Education and Applied Psychology. 2015;**3**:62-65

[14] Moskvina NV, Moskvin VA. Hemispheric asymmetry and features communication processes in sport psychology. European Journal of Education and Applied Psychology. 2015;**3**:59-62

[15] Moskvin VA, Moskvina NV, Shumova NS, Kovalevski AG. Tendency to risk and impulsiveness at students of sports university. Austrian Journal of Humanities and Social Sciences. 2015;**7-8**:80-84. DOI: 10.18411/d-2016-045

[16] Moskvin VA, Moskvina NV, Shumova NS, Kovalevski AG. Control over the actions in sports psychology. Austrian Journal of Humanities and

Social Sciences. 2015;**7-8**:84-86. DOI: 10.18411/d-2016-046

[17] Kuhl J, Schapkin S, Gusev A. A theory of volitional inhibition and an empirical test: Individual differences in the topography of ERP patterns for action-versus state oriented processing of emotional words. Forschungsberichte aus der Universität Osnabrück. 1994;**99**:1-52

[18] Moskvin VA, Moskvina NV, Shumova NS. Volitional regulation and features of motivation young players. European Journal of Education and Applied Psychology. 2016;**1**:59-62

[19] Moskvin VA, Moskvina KV. Sport managers goal-setting and psychological timing abilities. Theory and Practice of Physical Culture. 2017;**1**:38-39

[20] Golovakha EI, Kronik AA. Psychological Time of Personality. Kiev: Naukova Dumka; 1984. 207 p. (in Russian)

[21] Moskvin VA, Moskvina NV. Asymmetry and individual characteristics of strong-willed regulation teenage athletes. Austrian Journal of Humanities and Social Sciences. 2016;(5-6):22-24. DOI: 10.20534/AJH-16-5.6-22-24

[22] Moskvin VA, Moskvina NV, Tsangl N. Personal characteristics and motivation achievements of success in teenagers-figurers in connection with the peculiarities of asymmetry. European Science Review. 2017;**7-8**:90-91

[23] Rubinstein SL. Basics of General Psychology. 4th ed. Saint-Petersburg: Piter; 2000. 720 p. (in Russian). ISBN 5-314-00016-4

[24] Miller LI. Predicting relapse and recovery in alcoholism and addiction neuropsychology: Personality and cognitive style. Journal of Substance Abuse Treatment. 1991;**8**:277-291

[25] Moskvin V, Moskvina N. Individual peculiarities of students with manifestations of Internet addiction. European Science Review. 2018;(7-8):205-207

Chapter 5

Exercise Training and Cardiac Remodeling

Dayanne Borges, Suzilene Ormond, Murilo Nogueira, Keemilyn Silva and Jeeser Almeida

Abstract

The exercise training promotes functional and structural changes on several systems, including cardiovascular, resulting in physiological modifications responsible for maintaining variables such as cardiac output, preservation of blood flow, and the metabolic demand required in different sports. Recently, cardiac remodeling has been studied in order to broaden knowledge about the effects of physical training on cardiovascular characteristics in different populations. However, the adaptive responses inherent in exercise on cardiac remodeling seem to be influenced by other variables relevant to training, regulatory systems, and population specificity. Thus, this chapter aimed to elucidate the adaptive hypertrophic changes caused by physical exercise.

Keywords: physiological hypertrophy, physical exercise, hypertension, cardiac adaptation, sports

1. Introduction

The leading causes of death are due to cardiovascular disease (CVD), contributing substantially to increased health expenditure in several countries [1]. Thus, physical inactivity, obesity, smoking, and diabetes mellitus increased the risk for CVD [1]. Currently, sedentarism has been recognized as a primary risk factor, and physical exercise is associated with a decreased mortality rate from coronary artery disease [2]. Thus, a sedentary lifestyle is characterized as any waking behavior whose energy expenditure is less than 1.5 METs (metabolic equivalent), sitting, reclining, or lying down. This behavior differs from physical inactivity, which the individual does not perform moderate-vigorous physical activities [3].

Among the cardiovascular benefits of exercise, it is possible to observe blood pressure reductions, resting bradycardia, and greater efficiency of the cardiovascular system [4]. Also, cardioprotective factors are observed with exercise training such as the reduction of the magnitude of myocardial infarction [5], through different mechanisms, such as reduction of the inflammatory process, molecular regulation, as well as control of the pathological cardiac hypertrophy [5]. However, not every exercise stimulus promotes the same responses. Thus, it is necessary to know how much and what type of exercise should be applied to generate cardioprotective effects. For the prescription of exercises, it is essential to emphasize the variables that make up the activity: the FITT (frequency, intensity, type, and time) [6].

Aerobic exercise is considered a strategy for the prevention/treatment of arterial hypertension in reducing the risk of cardiovascular disease. The intensity of these exercises ranges from 40 to 60% of VO_{2max} or 11 to 14 of the perceived effort (Borg Scale). Current studies show that reductions in blood pressure by aerobic exercise are directly linked to intensity, so more vigorous activity may result in more significant reductions in blood pressure [6]. Frequency can range from 3 to 7 days a week [7, 8], and it is recommended to use large muscle groups, lasting 30–60 min [6]. Besides, several studies using resistance training (RT) as an intervention proposal are performed. Recent data indicate that RT has antihypertensive effects and can be used as a treatment strategy when combining with aerobic exercise [9, 10].

Consequently, exercise adaptations result in structural and physiological changes imposed on the heart. In this sense, cardiac remodeling occurs in different situations, which may be beneficial or harmful and widely studied in several aspects. Therefore, the purpose of this chapter is to review the aspects of cardiac remodeling associated with physical exercise.

2. Effects of exercise training in the arterial hypertension

For the past two decades, aerobic exercise (AE) has been used as a non-pharmacological therapy for cardiovascular disease control [11]. During an acute session of aerobic exercise, it is possible to verify the increase of specific cardiovascular parameters, such as cardiac output and blood pressure [12]. Interestingly, after the session, the values return to normal. However, blood pressure may fall below pre-exercise values; a phenomenon called post-exercise hypotension [13]. Additionally, aerobic training promotes significant changes in cardiovascular parameters. Long-term moderate-intense exercise promotes a reduction in arterial stiffness [14], a reduction in blood pressure [15], and an increase in cardiac efficiency [16]. Similarly, strength training is also helpful in lowering blood pressure as well as improving cardiovascular function [17].

Previous studies have shown that aerobic exercise causes structural and functional adaptations in the cardiovascular system [18, 19]. Thus, the heart has an essential morphological adaptation, characterized by an increase in the ventricular cavity, which is necessary for the more excellent supply of oxygen and nutrients [20]. The vascular system presents significant changes, such as increased vascular density due to the formation of new blood capillaries, associated with a higher vasodilator capacity [20]. RT has been well used to increase muscle strength, power, and endurance. However, it is essential to highlight how these effects are related to cardiovascular health in healthy individuals or those with CVD. Although RT is encouraged, the evidence is still controversial. However, evidence demonstrates a significant blood pressure reduction in unmedicated and medicated hypertensive patients [21].

Regarding the intensity of exercise, this may influence cardiovascular responses [22]. However, an optimal intensity for cardioprotection is not yet known [5]. In healthy individuals, cardiovascular changes seem to be more significant when subjected to the most intense effort [23]. Although high intensities have shown important outcomes for cardiovascular health, such as improved endothelial function, individuals with CVD need greater care in the assessment and prescription of intense exercise [5].

Arterial hypertension (AH) is considered as a major risk factor for diseases such as stroke and acute myocardial infarction [24]. SAH is diagnosed in individuals with sustained systolic blood pressure > 140 mmHg and/or diastolic blood pressure > 90 mm Hg [25]. The high prevalence of hypertension is related to non-modifiable factors such as ethnicity, gender, genetic factors, as well as modifiable environmental factors such as eating habits, physical activity level, smoking, and alcohol use, among others [24]. However pharmacological strategies for the treatment of hypertension are effective in controlling the disease, side effects, and health-care expenses which are considered relevant problems. In this sense, physical exercise has been considered as one of the most important and efficient strategies for non-pharmacological control of hypertension [26, 27].

Among the potential effects of exercise on hypertensive patients, post-exercise hypotension is of clinical relevance because it indicates a reduction in the progression of cardiovascular disease, and low resting BP values are associated with reduced risk of death [28]. Interestingly, hypertensive individuals have more significant reductions in blood pressure when compared to non-hypertensive individuals, both acutely and chronically [29, 30]. Besides, it has recently been proposed that acute response may be able to predict the responsiveness of hypertensive individuals to chronic exercise [31].

Exercise recommendations for hypertension treatment and prevention are based on existing evidence and are continually updated [32]. Thus, aerobic, resistance, and combined exercise present as effective alternatives (90–150 min per week at moderate intensity) [33]. Besides, other alternative strategies such as tai chi chuan, yoga, and even Kaatsu training have shown promising results, but due to the low body of evidence, they were considered limited to include the new recommendations [34, 35]. A randomized controlled trial (RCT) of 207 hypertensive subjects showed that 120 minutes of walking at moderate intensity without dietary control twice a week was able to reduce cardiovascular disease [36]. Also, during controlled eating, moderate aerobic exercise reduced blood pressure, total cholesterol levels, medication use, and the risk of cardiovascular events [37].

However, high-intensity interval training (HIIT) in cardiovascular responses in hypertensive patients has been increasingly discussed [15]. Therefore, another RCT with 245 hypertensive men (45–70 years) showed that 8 weeks of interval training performed at intensities of 60–78% (heart rate reserve—HRR) 3 times a week was able to promote a decreasing effect in reducing blood pressure and promote an increase in high-density lipoprotein (HDL) levels, improving lipid profile [38]. Additionally, a protocol using higher intensities (85–90% of HRR) is equally effective in promoting hypotensive effect in elderly hypertensive individuals, besides promoting increased nitric oxide, and appeals to important hemodynamic modulators [39]. RT is part of the recommendation for treatment and prevention of hypertension. Recently, a systematic meta-analysis review showed that RT, performed 3 times a week, with loads of 40–80% of 1 maximal repetition (MR), can lower blood pressure in individuals with high blood pressure [40]. Thus, RT has been a valuable alternative or complementary treatment to reduce blood pressure levels.

3. Characteristics of cardiac remodeling: effects of exercise training

The myocardium is primarily composed of myocytes, vessels, and interstitial collagen matrix. Changes in the composition of these compartments reflect the process of cardiac remodeling that is closely associated with cardiac dysfunction [41]. Cardiac hypertrophy is more often related to these events, and according to the type of hypertrophy (physiological or pathological), different models of it are observed, with their signaling pathways.

Cardiac remodeling can be defined as the set of cardiac molecular, cellular, and interstitial modifications that will be clinically displayed by changes in cavity diameter, mass (hypertrophy or atrophy), geometry (evidenced by wall thickness and heart shape), in response to a given stimulus, which may be aggression, such as areas with fibrosis and scarring observed in infarction [42] or even by adaptation, which is a physiological process, such as enlargement of the ventricular cavity of long-distance runners (eg marathon runners) [43–45]. The sequence of pathological events begins with aggressions to the cardiac tissue that maybe through reduction of myocyte changes in the energy system, pressure overload, and volume overload, among other factors. From one or a combination of these episodes, remodeling is a cascade of genetic, biochemical, molecular, cellular, and structural changes that most often culminate in ventricular dysfunction resulting in heart failure [46–48].

Myocytes perform the contractile function of the myocardium, and their preservation is fundamental since most of them are not capable of multiplication. Myocyte reduction can occur by three mechanisms: autophagy, apoptosis, and necrosis. New evidence indicates that for the latter, there is a confluence of mechanisms, and their close relationship is called necroptosis [49]. Autophagy, on the other hand, maybe adaptive or deleterious, depending on the context of protein balance. Fibrosis, observed in acute post-myocardial infarction situations, is a response to myocyte death since, after cardiac signaling for the removal of dead myocytes, cardiac fibroblasts secrete proteins such as collagen I to form a scar and prevent rupture of the myocardium cardiac wall. This condition, considered as remodeling, continues in response to ventricular wall stress, so we have another event called myocyte hypertrophy. This effect leads to increases in final systolic and diastolic volume and reduction in ejection fraction [50].

Energy metabolism and oxidative stress are factors potentially responsible for cardiac remodeling. The imbalance between oxygen supply and consumption, including decreased free fatty acids and increased glucose utilization, may contribute to lower energy availability for ATPase proteins, favoring the generation of reactive oxygen species (ROS), resulting in all the consequences of oxidative stress [51–53]. Lipid peroxidation, DNA damage, fibroblast proliferation, metalloproteinase activation, apoptosis stimulation, changes in proteins responsible for calcium transit, and activation of signaling pathways for hypertrophy are conditions involved in oxidative stress which is implied in the oxidative stress cardiac remodeling process due to cellular signaling and imbalances in homeostasis. In short, ROS directly influence contractile function from the modification of central proteins to the excitation-contraction. Continuous pressure overload promotes the addition of sarcomeres in parallel, that is, it promotes the increase in ventricular wall thickness, called concentric hypertrophy, which can be observed in advanced systemic arterial hypertension and aortic valve stenosis. On the other hand, volume overload (e.g., valve insufficiency) results in serial sarcomere increase, called eccentric hypertrophy [54], present in cases of acute myocardial infarction [55].

Regarding the pathological processes of concentric hypertrophy, muscle thickening hinders capillary filling in the deepest regions of the myocardium, specifically the subendocardium, which impairs the maintenance of blood flow. About eccentric hypertrophy, the increase in mass occurs with a predominance of increased intracavitary dimensions with less expression of myocardial thickening, causing cardiac fiber disarrangement and alteration in the angle between them, with loss of spiral architecture of the myocardial fibers, associated with a contractile deficit of the ventricle [55]. There is a blood damping in the cardiac chambers, decreasing the irrigation of peripheral tissues [56].

Regarding the process of physiological hypertrophy, both eccentric and concentric, the stimuli are similar to the process presented in serious pathologies (e.g., pressure and volume overload). However, what define the ventricular geometry pattern presented during remodeling are the characteristics inherent to the stimulus received, in which, in physiological cases, there are no functional damages to the cardiovascular system. Even more, adaptations from exercise can be beneficial in improving heart function. Hence, the physiological adaptations occur from physical exercise, for example, depending on the type of exercise (e.g., running and strength training) of volume, intensity, and frequency. Regarding the benefits of regular aerobic exercise practice, there is a higher blood volume ejection due to increased ejection force or higher ventricular filling, thus reducing the resting heart rate.

Diverse molecular pathways are associated with exercise-induced cardiac remodeling. However, the gene pathway (IGF-1) is well characterized and evidenced in the literature [57], due to the increase in cardiomyocytes in response to aerobic exercise [58]. However, cardiac remodeling in response to aerobic training is dependent to PI3K pathway activation and AKT phosphorylation [59]. Interestingly, short-term, aerobic training (4 weeks) can reprogram cardiac remodeling through AKT activity [60]. Additionally, in both animal and human models, exercise can attenuate the deleterious effects of aging [61, 62].

The role of miRNAs is of fundamental importance in the cardiac remodeling process [55, 63] mainly associated with exercise training [64, 65], due to their participation in left ventricular hypertrophy in aerobic exercise. Also, HIIT protocols show miRNA expression in cardiac hypertrophy [55]. Thus, exercise is an essential factor in identifying miRNA signatures associated with cardiac remodeling. MiRNA-29 targets the collagen gene, which increases with the induction of physical exercise, reducing collagen I and III, resulting in better ventricular function [66]. Also, miRNA-29 reduces collagen fibrosis and attenuates the deleterious effects of cardiovascular disease [67]. Therefore, although miRNAs and genes are closely related to the cardiac remodeling process, other factors are also important, such as proteomics and metabolomics. So many pieces still need to be fitted into this cardiac puzzle.

4. Conclusions

Regardless of the type of stimulus imposed by exercise, the key point to ensuring positive myocardial adaptations is in the balance of training manipulation variables (frequency, intensity, and volume) as well as the nature of the modality chosen. Considering the intensity variable, which is widely investigated, it is clear that while low-intensity aerobic exercise improves cardiac remodeling in adult rats by reducing the size of the left atrium and the left ventricular (LV) posterior wall thickness, high-intensity aerobic exercise presents inverse responses, with increased left ventricular mass and LV posterior wall thickness. Dynamic exercise (running), which requires a continuous increase in cardiac function and contractility, differs from powerlifting which requires high blood pressure and a greater need for oxygen perfusion to skeletal muscles. This explains the ability of the circulatory system to differentiate exercise types according to different hematological stresses.

The responses related to the type of exercise are diverse, as they are interpreted from different experimental and clinical designs. Still, it is critical to search for research to assess the chronic effects of exercise, especially at the molecular level to find strategies for the prevention and treatment of cardiovascular disease. Perspectives point to the integration of studies involving immune response in the brain and heart in order to contribute to the understanding and longitudinal follow-up of several modalities, including the determination of the threshold of optimal internal and external stimulus loads to avoid cardiac toxicity, which leads to pathological cardiac remodeling, also considering the screening of individuals at risk.

Acknowledgements

This chapter integrates the result of all the support given by the Exercise, Nutrition, Health and Performance Research Group–PENSARE, Federal University of Mato Grosso do Sul through the project MEDALHA (Multiprofessionalism in Sport: Determinants of High Performance and Longevity of Athletes) (https://www.projetomedalha.org/home/) which provides multidisciplinary and interinstitutional care to athletes from Mato Grosso do Sul, analyzing health and physical performance through tests and exams with reputable professionals.

Notes/thanks/other declarations

This chapter discloses the experiences of the group of teachers/researchers of the Faculty of Physical Education of Federal University of Mato Grosso do Sul which will be of great use to all students and health professionals interested in deepening their knowledge in the field of exercise cardiology.

Appendices and nomenclature

AKT	protein kinase B: is a threonine kinase that plays a critical role in cellular growth and survival
ATPase	an enzyme that catalyzes the breakdown of adenosine triphosphate (ATP) into adenosine diphosphate (ADP) and a free phosphate ion
IGF-1	insulin-like growth factor 1: peptide that acts on glucose and amino acid uptake into cells
HDL	high-density lipoprotein: is a strong inverse predictor of cardiovascular events
HIIT	high-intensity interval training: is an enhanced form of interval training involving brief, high-intensity, anaerobic exercise (ranging from 85–250% VO_{2max} for 6 s–4 min) separated by brief but slightly longer bouts of low-intensity aerobic rest (ranging from 20–40% VO_{2max} for 10 s–5 min)
HRR	heart rate reserve: it is the term used to describe the difference between the maximum HR (measured or calculated) and the basal (or resting) HR. It is used as an intensity control variable in aerobic exercises. The greater the difference between maximal HR and basal HR1, the higher the reserve HR, and the greater its potential to train at different intensities
MR	maximal repetition: used as a measure of muscle strength, whether in physical preparation, sports training, physical rehabilitation, or scientific research
METs	metabolic equivalent: Is equivalent to sufficient energy for an individual to remain at rest, represented in the literature by oxygen consumption (VO_2) of approximately 3.5 ml/kg/min. When expressing energy expenditure in METs, the number of times the resting metabolism was multiplied during an activity is expressed
MiRNAs	they are 19–25 molecules nonprotein-coding nucleotides that act as potent posttranscriptional regulators of gene expression in plants and animals
PI3K	phosphatidylinositol 3-kinase: constitutes a family of evolutionarily conserved lipid kinases that regulate a vast array of

	fundamental cellular responses, including proliferation, adhesion, cell size, and protection from apoptosis
RT	resistance training: resistance training is defined as an exercise that involves the participant exerting effort against their body weight or external resistance
ROS	reactive oxygen species: they are unstable and extremely reactive molecules capable of transforming other molecules with which they collide. The EROs are generated in large quantities during oxidative stress, a condition in which molecules such as proteins, carbohydrates, lipids, and nucleic acids are affected

Author details

Dayanne Borges[1], Suzilene Ormond[1], Murilo Nogueira[1], Keemilyn Silva[1] and Jeeser Almeida[1,2]*

1 Exercise and Nutrition Research in Health and Sports Performance–PENSARE, Health and Development in the Midwest Region, Federal University of Mato Grosso do Sul, Campo Grande, Brazil

2 Graduate Program in Movement Sciences, Federal University of Mato Grosso do Sul, Campo Grande, Brazil

*Address all correspondence to: jeeser@gmail.com

References

[1] SSAC. Sociedade Sul-Americana de Cardiologia. Diretriz Sul-Americana de Prevenção e Reabilitação Cardiovascular [Internet]. 2015. Available from: http://www.scielo.br/pdf/abc/v103n2s1/pt_0066-782X-abc-103-02-s1-0001.pdf [Accessed: 18 July 2019]

[2] Paudel S, Owen AJ, Owusu-Addo E, Smith BJ. Physical activity participation and the risk of chronic diseases among south Asian adults: A systematic review and meta-analysis. Scientific Reports. 2019;**9**:1-12. DOI: 10.1038/s41598-019-46154-3

[3] Lavie CJ, Ozemek C, Carbone S, Katzmarzyk PT, Blair SN. Sedentary behavior, exercise, and cardiovascular health. Circulation Research. 2019;**124**:799-815. DOI: 10.1161/circresaha.118.312669

[4] De Brito LC, Fecchio RY, Peçanha T, Lima A, Halliwill J, Forjaz CLM. Recommendations in post-exercise hypotension: Concerns, best practices and interpretation. International Journal of Sports Medicine. 2019;**40**:487-497. DOI: 10.1055/a-0938-4415

[5] Chowdhury MA, Sholl HK, Sharrett MS, Haller ST, Cooper CC, Gupta R, et al. Exercise and cardioprotection: A natural defense against lethal myocardial ischemia–reperfusion injury and potential guide to cardiovascular prophylaxis. Journal of Cardiovascular Pharmacology and Therapeutics. 2018;**24**:18-30. DOI: 10.1177/1074248418788575

[6] ACSM, American College of Sports Medicine. Exercise for the Prevention and Treatment of Hypertension–Implications and Application [Internet]. 2019. Available from: https://www.acsm.org/blog-detail/acsm-certified-blog/2019/02/27/exercise-hypertension-prevention-treatment [Accessed: 15 July 2019]

[7] Rêgo ML, Cabral DA, Costa EC, Fontes EB. Physical exercise for individuals with hypertension: It is time to emphasize its benefits on the brain and cognition. Clinical Medicine Insights Cardiology. 2019;**13**:1-10. DOI: 10.1177/1179546819839411

[8] Börjesson M, Onerup A, Lundqvist S, Dahlöf B. Physical activity and exercise lower blood pressure in individuals with hypertension: Narrative review of 27 RCTs. British Journal of Sports Medicine. 2016;**50**:356-361. DOI: 10.1136/bjsports-2015-095786

[9] Cornelissen VA, Fagard RH, Coeckelberghs E, Vanhees L. Impact of resistance training on blood pressure and other cardiovascular risk factors. Hypertension. 2011;**58**:950-958. DOI: 10.1161/hypertensionaha.111.177071

[10] Nascimento DDC, da Silva CR, Valduga R, Saraiva B, de Sousa Neto IV, Vieira A, et al. Blood pressure response to resistance training in hypertensive and normotensive older women. Clinical Interventions in Aging. 2018;**13**:541-553. DOI: 10.2147/cia.s157479

[11] Gary RA, Cress ME, Higgins MK, Smith AL, Dunbar SB. Combined aerobic and resistance exercise program improves task performance in patients with heart failure. Arquives Physical Medicine and Rehabilitation. 2011;**92**:1371-1381. DOI: 10.1016/j.apmr.2011.02.022

[12] Brum PC, Forjaz CLM, Tinucci T, Negrão CE. Adaptações agudas e crônicas do exercício físico no sistema cardiovascular. Revista Paulista de Educação Física. 2004;**18**:21-31

[13] Shiotsu Y, Watanabe Y, Tujii S, Yanagita M. Effect of exercise order of combined aerobic and resistance training on arterial stiffness in older men. Experimental Gerontology.

2018;**1**:27-34. DOI: 10.1016/j.exger.2018.06.020

[14] Alvim RO, Santos PCJL, Bortolotto LA, Mill JG, Pereira AC. Rigidezarterial: Aspectosfisiopatológicos e genéticos. International Journal of Cardiovascular Sciences. 2017;**30**:433-441. DOI: 10.5935/2359-4802.20170053

[15] Boutcher YN, Boutcher SH. Exercise intensity and hypertension: what's new? Journal of Human Hypertension. 2016;**31**:1-8. DOI: 10.1038/jhh.2016.62

[16] Cavalcante PAM, Perilhão MS, Da Silva AA, Serra AJ, Figueira Júnior A, Bocalini DS. Cardiac remodeling and physical exercise: A brief review about concepts and adaptations. International Journal of Sports Science. 2016;**6**:52-61. DOI: 10.5923/j.sports.20160602.06

[17] Gerage AM, Cyrino ES, Schiavoni D, Nakamura FY, Ronque ERV, Gurjão ALD, et al. Efeito de 16 semanas de treinamento com pesos sobre a pressão arterial em mulheres normotensas e não-treinadas. Revista Brasileira de Medicina do Esporte. 2007;**13**:361-365. DOI: 10.1590/S1517-86922007000600001

[18] Gunadi JW, Tarawan VM, Setiawan I, Lesmana R, Wahyudianingsih R, Supratman U. Cardiac hypertrophy is stimulated by altered training intensity and correlates with autophagy modulation in male Wistar rats. BMC Sports Science, Medicine and Rehabilitation. 2019;**10**: 1-9. DOI: 10.1186/s13102-019-0121-0

[19] Lavie CJ, Arena R, Swift DL, Johannsen NM, Sui X, Lee DC, et al. Exercise and the cardiovascular system: Clinical science and cardiovascular outcomes. Circulation Research. 2015;**3**:207-219. DOI: 10.1161/CIRCRESAHA.117.305205

[20] Nystoriak MA, Bhatnagar A. Cardiovascular effects and benefits of exercise. Frontiers in Cardiovascular Medicine. 2018;**5**:1-11. DOI: 10.3389/fcvm.2018.00135

[21] MacDonald HV, Johnson BT, Huedo-Medina TB, Livingston J, Forsyth KC, Kraemer WJ, et al. Dynamic resistance training as stand-alone antihypertensive lifestyle therapy: A meta-analysis. Journal of the American Heart Association. 2016;**5**:1-15. DOI: 10.1161/JAHA.116.003231

[22] Tsukamoto H, Suga T, Takenaka S, Tanaka D, Takeuchi T, Hamaoka T, et al. Greater impact of acute high-intensity interval exercise on post-exercise executive function compared to moderate-intensity continuous exercise. Physiology & Behavior. 2016;**155**:224-230. DOI: 10.1016/j.physbeh.2015.12.021

[23] Golbini S, Laher I. Exercise and the cardiovascular system. Cardiology Research and Practice. 2012;**2012**:1-5. DOI: 10.1155/2012/210852

[24] GBD 2013 Risk Factors Collaborators*. Global, regional, and national comparative risk assessment of 79 behavioural, environmental and occupational, and metabolic risks or clusters of risks in 188 countries, 1990-2013: A systematic analysis for the global burden of disease study 2013. Lancet. 2015;**386**:2287-2323. DOI: 10.1016/S0140-6736(15)00128-2

[25] Messerli FH, Williams B, Ritz E. Essential hypertension. Lancet. 2007;**370**:591-603. DOI: 10.1016/S0140-6736(07)61299-9

[26] Whelton PK, Carey RM, Aronow WS, Casey DE Jr, Collins KJ, Dennison Himmelfarb C, et al. 2017 ACC/AHA/AAPA/ABC/ACPM/AGS/APhA/ASH/ASPC/NMA/PCNA guideline for the prevention, detection, evaluation, and management of high blood pressure in adults: A report of the American College of Cardiology/American Heart Association task

force on clinical practice guidelines. Hypertension. 2018;**71**:1269-1324. DOI: 10.1161/HYP.0000000000000065

[27] Vagnoni E, Biavati GR, Felisatti M, Pomidori L. Moderating healthcare costs through an assisted physical activity programme. The International Journal of Health Planning and Manage. 2018;**33**:1146-1158. DOI: 10.1002/hpm.2596

[28] Hu G, Jousilahti P, Antikainen R, Tuomilehto J. Occupational, commuting, and leisure-time physical activity in relation to cardiovascular mortality among Finnish subjects with hypertension. American Journal of Hypertension. 2007;**20**:1242-1250. DOI: 10.1016/j.amjhyper.2007.07.015

[29] Ramirez-Jimenez M, Morales-Palomo F, Pallares JG, Mora-Rodriguez R, Ortega JF. Ambulatory blood pressure response to a bout of HIIT in metabolic syndrome patients. European Journal of Applied Physiology. 2017;**117**:1403-1411. DOI: 10.1007/s00421-017-3631

[30] Ramos RM, Coelho-Júnior HJ, Asano RY, Prado RCR, Silveira R, Urtado CB, et al. Impact of moderate aerobic training on physical capacities of hypertensive obese elderly. Gerontology & Geriatric Medicine. 2019;**5**:1-9. DOI: 10.1177/2333721419859691

[31] Wegmann M, Hecksteden A, Poppendieck W, Steffen A, Kraushaar J, Morsch A, et al. Postexercise hypotension as a predictor for long-term training-induced blood pressure reduction: A large-scale randomized controlled trial. Clinical Journal of Sport Medicine. 2018;**28**:509-515. DOI: 10.1097/JSM.0000000000000475

[32] Pescatello LS, Bloodgood B, Buchner D, Campbell W, Dietz S, DiPietro L, et al., for the 2018 Physical Activity Guidelines Advisory Committee. Physical activity to prevent and treat hypertension. Medicine and Science in Sports and Exercise. 2019;**51**:1314-1323. DOI: 10.1249/MSS.0000000000001943

[33] ASCM. In: Riebe D, Ehrman JK, Liguori G, Magal M, editors. ACSM Guidelines for Exercise Testing and Prescription 10th Edition. Philadelphia, PA: Wolters Kluwer Health; 2018. Available from: https://www.acsm.org/read-research/books/acsms-guidelines-for-exercise-testing-and-prescription [Accessed: 16 July 2019]

[34] Ciolac EG, Bocchi EA, Bortolotto LA, Carvalho VO, Greve JM, Guimarães GV. Effects of high-intensity aerobic interval training vs. moderate exercise on hemodynamic, metabolic and neuro-humoral abnormalities of young normotensive women at high familial risk for hypertension. Hypertension Research. 2010;**33**: 836-843. DOI: 10.1038/hr.2010.72

[35] Ciolac EG. High-intensity interval training and hypertension: Maximizing the benefits of exercise? American Journal of Cardiovascular Disease. 2012;**2**:102-110

[36] Arija V, Villalobos F, Pedret R, Vinuesa A, Jovani D, Pascual G, et al. Physical activity, cardiovascular health, quality of life and blood pressure control in hypertensive subjects: Randomized clinical trial. Health and Quality of Life Outcomes. 2018;**16**:1-11. DOI: 10.1186/s12955-018-1008-6

[37] Gorostegi-Anduaga I, Maldonado-Martín S, MartinezAguirre-Betolaza A, Corres P, Romaratezabala E, Whittaker AC, et al. Efects on cardiovascular risk scores and vascular age after aerobic exercise and nutritional intervention in sedentary and overweight/obese adults with primary hypertension: The EXERDIET-HTA randomized trial study. High Blood Pressure and Cardiovascular Prevention. 2018;**25**:361-368. DOI: 10.1007/s40292-018-0281-0

[38] Lamina S, Okoye GC. Therapeutic effect of a moderate intensity interval training program on the lipid profile in men with hypertension: A randomized controlled trial. Nigerian Journal of Clinical Practice. 2012;**15**:42-47. DOI: 10.4103/1119-3077.94096

[39] Izadi MR, Ghardashi Afousi A, Asvadi Fard M, Babaee Bigi MA. High-intensity interval training lowers blood pressure and improves apelin and NOx plasma levels in older treated hypertensive individuals. Journal of Physiology and Biochemistry. 2018;**74**:47-55. DOI: 10.1007/s13105-017-0602-0

[40] Costa EC, Hay JL, Kehler DS, Boreskie KF, Arora RC, Umpierre D, et al. Effects of high-intensity interval training versus moderate intensity continuous training on blood pressure in adults with pre-to established hypertension: A systematic review and meta-analysis of randomized trials. Sports Medicine. 2018;**48**:2127-2142. DOI: 10.1007/s40279-018-0944-y

[41] Weber KT. Targeting pathological remodeling–Concepts of cardioprotection and reparation. Circulation. 2000;**102**:1342-1345. DOI: 10.1161/01.CIR.102.12.1342

[42] Cohn JN, Ferrari R, Sharpe N. Cardiac remodeling-concepts and clinical implications: A consensus paper from an international forum on cardiac remodeling. Behalf of an International Forum on Cardiac Remodeling. Journal of the American College of Cardiology. 2000;**35**:569-582. DOI: 10.1016/s0735-1097(99)00630-0

[43] Ghorayeb N, Batlouni M, Pinto IMF, Dioguardi GS. Hipertrofia ventricular esquerda do atleta. Resposta adaptativa fisiológica do coração. Arquivos Brasileiros de Cardiologia. 2005;**85**:191-197. DOI: 10.1590/S0066-782X2005001600008

[44] Azevedo LF, Brum PC, Rosemblatt D, Perlingeiro Pde S, Barretto AC, Negrão CE, et al. Cardiac and metabolic characteristics in long distance runners of sport and exercise cardiology outpatient facility of a tertiary hospital. Arquivos Brasileiros de Cardiologia. 2007;**88**:17-25. DOI: 10.1590/s0066-782x2007000100003

[45] Kinoshita N, Katsukawa F, Yamazaki H. Modeling of longitudinal changes in left ventricular dimensions among female adolescent runners. PLoS One. 2015;**10**:1-14. DOI: 10.1371/journal.pone.0140573

[46] Zornoff LA, Paiva SA, Duarte DR, Spadaro J. Ventricular remodeling after myocardial infarction: Concepts and clinical implications. Arquivos Brasileiros de Cardiologia. 2009;**92**:157-164. DOI: 10.1590/s0066-782x2009000200013

[47] Swynghedauw B. Phenotypic plasticity of adult myocardium: Molecular mechanisms. The Journal of Experimental Biology. 2006;**209**:2320-2327. DOI: 10.1242/jeb.02084

[48] Heusch G, Libby P, Gersh B, Yellon D, Lopaschuk G, Opie L. Cardiovascular remodelling in coronary artery disease and heart failure. Lancet. 2014;**383**:1933-1943. DOI: 10.1016/S0140-6736(14)60107-0

[49] Burchfield JS, Xie M, Hill JA. Pathological ventricular remodeling: Mechanisms: Part 1 of 2. Circulation. 2013;**128**:388-400. DOI: 10.1161/CIRCULATIONAHA.113.001878

[50] Dorn GW. Novel pharmacotherapies to abrogate postinfarction ventricular remodeling. Nature Reviews. Cardiology. 2009;**6**:283-291. DOI: 10.1038/nrcardio.2009.12

[51] Campos DH, Leopoldo AS, Lima-Leopoldo AP, Nascimento AF, Oliveira-Junior SA, Silva DCT, et al.

Obesity preserves myocardial function during blockade of the glycolytic pathway. Arquivos Brasileiros de Cardiologia. 2014;**103**:330-337. DOI: 10.5935/abc.20140135

[52] Azevedo PS, Minicucci MF, Santos PP, Paiva SA, Zornoff LA. Energy metabolism in cardiac remodeling and heart failure. Cardiology in Review. 2013;**21**: 135-140. DOI: 10.1097/CRD. 0b013e318274956d

[53] Santos PP, Oliveira F, Ferreira VC, Polegato BF, Roscani MG, Fernandes AA, et al. The role of lipotoxicity in smoke cardiomyopathy. PLoS One. 2014;**9**:1-13. DOI: 10.1371/ journal.pone.0113739

[54] Matsubara LS, Narikawa S, Ferreira ALA, de PSAR, Zornoff LM, Matsubara BB. Remodelação miocárdica na sobrecarga crônica de pressão ou de volume no coração de ratos. Arquivos Brasileiros de Cardiologia. 2006;**86**:126-130. DOI: 10.1590/ S0066-782X2006000200008

[55] Da Silva ND Jr, Fernandes T, Soci UP, Monteiro AW, Phillips MI, de Oliveira EM. Swimming training in rats increases cardiac MicroRNA-126 expression and angiogenesis. Medicine and Science of Sports Exercise. 2012;**44**:1453-1462. DOI: 10.1249/ MSS.0b013e31824e8a36

[56] Seo DY, Kwak HB, Kim AH, Park SH, Heo JW, Kim HK, et al. Cardiac adaptation to exercise training in health and disease. Pflugers Arch. 23 Apr 2019. DOI: 10.1007/s00424-019-02266-3. [Epub ahead of print]

[57] Vega RB, Konhilas JP, Kelly DP, Leinwand LA. Molecular mechanisms underlying cardiac adaptation to exercise. Cell Metabolism. 2017;**25**:1012-1026. DOI: 10.1016/j. cmet.2017.04.025

[58] Neri Serneri GG, Boddi M, Modesti PA, Cecioni I, Coppo M, Padeletti L, et al. Increased cardiac sympathetic activity and insulin-like growth factor-I formation are associated with physiological hypertrophy in athletes. Circulation Research. 2001;**89**:977-982. DOI: 10.1161/ hh2301.100982

[59] McMullen JR, Shioi T, Huang WY, Zhang L, Tarnavski O, Bisping E, et al. The insulin-like growth factor 1 receptor induces physiological heart growth via the phosphoinositide 3-kinase(p110alpha) pathway. The Journal of Biological Chemistry. 2004;**279**:4782-4793. DOI: 10.1074/jbc. M310405200

[60] Wadley GD, Laker RC, McConell GK, Wlodek ME. Endurance training in early life results in long-term programming of heart mass in rats. Physiological Reports. 2016;**4**:1-14. DOI: 10.14814/phy2.12720

[61] Leosco D, Iaccarino G, Cipolletta E, De Santis D, Pisani E, Trimarco V, et al. Exercise restores beta-adrenergic vasorelaxation in aged rat carotid arteries. American Journal of Physiology. Heart and Circulatory Physiology. 2003;**285**:369-374. DOI: 10.1152/ajpheart.00019.2003

[62] Leosco D, Parisi V, Femminella GD, Formisano R, Petraglia L, Allocca E, et al. Effects of exercise training on cardiovascular adrenergic system. Frontiers in Physiology. 2013;**4**:1-7. DOI: 10.3389/fphys.2013.00348

[63] Fish JE, Santoro MM, Morton SU, Yu S, Yeh RF, Wythe JD, et al. miR-126 regulates angiogenic signaling and vascular integrity. Developmental Cell. 2008;**15**:272-284. DOI: 10.1016/j. devcel.2008.07.008

[64] Fernandes T, Hashimoto NY, Magalhães FC, Fernandes FB,

Casarini DE, Carmona AK, et al. Aerobic exercise training-induced left ventricular hypertrophy involves regulatory MicroRNAs, decreased angiotensin-converting enzyme-angiotensin II, and synergistic regulation of angiotensin-converting enzyme 2-angiotensin (1-7). Hypertension. 2011;**58**:182-189. DOI: 10.1161/HYPERTENSIONAHA.110.168252

[65] Soci UPR, Fernandes T, Barauna VG, Hashimoto NY, Mota GFA, Rosa KT, et al. Epigenetic control of exercise training-induced cardiac hypertrophy by miR-208. Clinical Science. 2016;**130**(22):2005-2015. DOI: 10.1042/CS20160480

[66] Soci UP, Fernandes T, Hashimoto NY, Mota GF, Amadeu MA, Rosa KT, et al. MicroRNAs 29 are involved in the improvement of ventricular compliance promoted by aerobic exercise training in rats. Physiological Genomics. 2011;**43**:665-673. DOI: 10.1152/physiolgenomics.00145.2010

[67] Melo SF, Fernandes T, Baraúna VG, Matos KC, Santos AA, Tucci PJ, et al. Expression of microRNA-29 and collagen in cardiac muscle after swimming training in myocardial-infarcted rats. Cellullar Physiology and Biochemistry. 2014;**33**:657-669. DOI: 10.1159/000358642

Chapter 6

Motives of Training and Sport Routine Highly Qualified Athletes of 5-a-Side Blind Football National Sport Team of Russia

Konstantin Popenko

Abstract

This article presents the results of studies on the motivation of highly qualified athletes involved in Paralympics sport football five-a-side, which was held at the international friendly tournament in Silvi Marina (Italy) in June 2018. The main factors determining the importance of results in achieving the results are physical and mental stresses corresponding to critical values. The study of sports motivation of qualified Paralympics football players of the national team of the Russian Federation began with the definition of a list of motives for playing football five-a-side (sports of the blind). Analysis and generalization of literary sources made it possible to form an extended circle of motivation, and interviewing and questioning current athletes and coaches, allowed to determine the list of motives of highly qualified athletes, included in the questionnaire for study. The study involved active athletes of the youth and main staff of the Russian national team. Football players represented three regions: Moscow, Moscow Region, and the Republic of Mari El. In total, 13 respondents took part in the survey. The data obtained were statistically processed using the method of average values (calculations were performed using the standard Microsoft Excel for Windows software package).

Keywords: Paralympics sport, five-a-side blind football, motivation, national sport team of Russia, highly qualified athletes, sports training management

1. Introduction

The development of adaptive sports in Russia at the territorial level is not evenly. Often several cities, regions or republics cultivate only a single species; therefore, athletes from two or three regions form the country's national sport team.

The problems of developing Paralympic futsal (blind sports) remain without due attention, and only a few regions are actively involved in resolving them. One of these problems is the methodological content of the sports training programs for the sports reserve for five-a-side blind football. The program should include best practices in training the national team of the country, be applied in nature. The normative and methodological documentation for this Paralympics discipline is not informative or completely absent today, which means that there are no guidelines for the development of sports training programs both in the country as a whole and in the regions separately. The current methodological and used material is formal and borrowed from other sports, often intended for healthy athletes.

The study draws the attention of trainers and specialists about the need to apply a scientific and methodological approach to managing the training process not only in the preparation of high-class players of the national team, but also in the sports reserve at earlier stages of preparation.

2. Motives of training and sport routine highly qualified athletes of five-a-side blind football national sport team of Russia

In recent decades, the sport of the blind in the world is developing at a rapid pace. In the Russian Federation, according to the All-Russian Register of Sports, the sport of the blind includes 203 sports disciplines in 9 sports included in the program of the Paralympic Games (cycling tandem, goal ball, judo, athletics, swimming, futsal, skiing, ski racing, biathlon) [1].

The number of sporting events, both international and national, is increasing annually, and the number of participants is growing. With close cooperation between the federations, state, and public organizations of the disabled, significant work is underway to develop various sports for the visually impaired. Experienced coaches train disabled athletes (hereinafter referred to as athletes) for the national teams of Russia and the Russian Paralympic team. Together with the Russian Ministry of Sports, national and international competitions of various levels are organized and held. Particular attention is paid to working with children from sponsored boarding schools who undergo rehabilitation in clubs and sections [2].

Moreover, according to the President of the Blind Sports Federation Abramova Lidia Pavlovna, there is a tendency in Russia to uneven development sports disciplines of the sport of the blind at the regional level. Five-a-side blind football did not pass this trend, despite the fact that, along with athletics, swimming and ski racing, it is the most popular sport among blind and visually impaired people [3, 4].

So, in Moscow, Moscow Region, Nizhny Novgorod Region, the Republic of Dagestan, the Republic of Mari El and the Republic of Tatarstan, the Khabarovsk Territory, much attention is paid to the development of 5×5 (B1) indoor football (blind sports) (hereinafter referred to as five-a-side blind football), then in other regions this is not observed. Today, problems associated with the training of qualified coaching personnel, the lack of a special methodology for training athletes and insufficient provision of scientific and methodological literature for the preparation of a sports reserve continue to remain unresolved [5, 6].

In this regard, for a more effective development of five-a-side blind football, it is necessary to resolve problems associated with the insufficient development of a scientifically based system for training coaches and athletes in this sport. It also requires refinement and improvement of the methodological content of the content of sports training programs, which should be based on many years of experience in training highly qualified Paralympic futsal players, players of the national team of the Russian Federation, demonstrating high results at international competitions in recent years. The sport of the highest achievements is associated with high social significance, a public assessment of successes and failures, publicity, interaction with the media. In stressful situations of competitive activity, under equal training conditions, when physical and mental stress reaches a critical value, the level of motivation and personal characteristics are crucial in achieving the result [7].

A highly qualified athlete enters into complex interactions and relationships with the chosen sport, which in turn presents special specific requirements for physical qualities, behavioral habits, personal characteristics, and his sports motivation. Therefore, it is so important for a high-class athlete, along with full compliance with the requirements of the sport, exceptional sports motivation, which will allow him to realize his potential, achieve high sports results, and become one of the best athletes in his country.

In parallel with this study, we carried out work on the study of the main motives for playing five-a-side blind football of qualified Italian football players [8].

Prerequisites for the work were the thesis based on scientific and methodological literature and coaching experience, according to which not all athletes who are gifted by nature achieve significant success. Therefore, the determination of the motivation features of highly qualified athletes can help the trainer not only in planning sports training with the optimal amount of training and competition load, but also in creating pedagogical conditions for implementing this training program.

Among the active domestic Russian researchers of motives, motives of sports activities in individual sports, issues of motivation in adaptive sports, A. A. Antonov, E. G. Babushkin, G. D. Babushkin, G. D. Gorbunov, G. B. Gorskaya, E. P. Ilyin, N. D. Ivanova, T. E. Kazakova, A. V. Korneva, M. A. Korneva, E. B. Kuzmin, A. S. Makhov, L. R. Makina, A. N. Nikolaev, E. A. Osokina, E. Yu. Pelikh, R. A. Piloyan, P. A. Rudik, O. M. Rumyantseva, O. G. Rysakova, A. V. Shaboltas, O. N. Stepanova, Zhabakov T. V., A. V. Zhalilov and E. G. Znamenskaya [2, 9–15].

Despite the great attention to sports motivation by scientists and experts in the field of physical culture and sports, an analysis of domestic Russian scientific literature showed that the motivation of high-class athletes has not been studied enough. Moreover, the study of the motives of sports activity of athletes in team types of adaptive sports was not carried out at all before.

2.1 Research methods and organization

The study of sports motivation of qualified Paralympic football players of the national team of the Russian Federation began with the definition of a list of motives for playing five-a-side blind football. Analysis and generalization of literary sources allowed us to form an expanded circle of motivation [2, 10, 14, 15], and interviewing and questioning existing athletes and coaches that are part of the country's youth and main Paralympic futsal team, allowed us to determine the list of motives of highly qualified athletes, included in the questionnaire for this study (**Table 1**).

Respondents were asked to indicate the degree (point) of importance of the proposed motives on a 10-point scale (1 point-minimum, 10 points-maximum). Moreover, depending on the degree of significance of the motive, expressed in points, the answers were divided into groups: 9–10 points: "extremely important", 7–8 points: "very important", 5–6 points: "pretty important", 3–4 points: "not very important", 1–2 points: "absolutely not important".

The questionnaire was conducted in June 2018 during the period in which the international friendly football tournament 5 × 5 (B1) (sport of the blind) was held in Silvi Marina (Italy). The study involved active athletes of the youth and main staff of the Russian national team. Football players represented three regions: Moscow, Moscow Region and the Republic of Mari El. In total, 13 respondents took part in the survey. The data obtained were statistically processed using the method of average values (calculations were performed using the standard Microsoft Excel for Windows software package).

2.2 Results and its discussion

Questioning of Russian highly qualified Paralympic futsal players showed that four motives are not significant and are classified in the category "Absolutely not

Dear colleagues!

The research group of state-financed institution of the Republic of Mari El "Sports-adaptive school of Paralympic reserve" (Yoshkar-Ola) and the Russian state social University (Moscow) addresses to you. Could you please answer the questionnaire?

The questionnaire

Please give us some information about yourself: your age is ________.

Place of residence (country, city) ________________________.

Below you can find a list of motives of qualified athletes to practice five-a-side blind football, evaluate the importance of each of them on a 10-point scale.

9–10	**7–8**	**5–6**	**3–4**	**1–2**
Extremely important	Very important	Quite important	Not very important	It does not matter

Write down the chosen rate

No	**Мотивы квалифицированных спортсменов**	**Motives of qualified athletes**	**Rate**
1	Постоянно находишься в состоянии физического или эмоционального напряжения	You are always in a state of physical or emotional stress	10 9 8 7 6 5 4 3 2 1
2	Мотивом является достижение успеха, которое постоянно подкрепляется промежуточными достижениями: гол, победа, медаль	Your motive is achievement of success which is constantly supported by intermediate achievements: a goal, a victory, a medal	10 9 8 7 6 5 4 3 2 1
3	Развивает характер, психические и физические качества	Develops character, mental and physical qualities	10 9 8 7 6 5 4 3 2 1
4	Совершенствование личностных качеств таких, как выдержка, воля, взаимопомощь, терпение	Improvement of personal qualities such as endurance, will, mutual assistance, patience	10 9 8 7 6 5 4 3 2 1
5	Нравится сам процесс спортивной подготовки и её составляющие компоненты: тренировки, сборы, товарищеские игры, контрольные соревнования и т.д	You like the process of sports training and its components: training, training camps, friendly games, control competitions, etc.	10 9 8 7 6 5 4 3 2 1
6	Одобрение и поддержка со стороны значимых для меня людей: родственников, друзей, других близких людей	Approval and support from important people for me: relatives, friends, other close people	10 9 8 7 6 5 4 3 2 1
7	Способ удовлетворения потребности в новых ощущениях, и стремление доказать, что способен на большее	A way to meet the need for new sensations, and the desire to prove that you are capable to do more	10 9 8 7 6 5 4 3 2 1
8	Возможность проявить себя, свои способности, умения, личностные качества	The opportunity to express yourself, your abilities, skills, personal qualities	10 9 8 7 6 5 4 3 2 1
9	Возможность выплеснуть эмоции, снять нервное и психическое напряжение	The ability to throw out emotions, relieve nervous and mental tension	10 9 8 7 6 5 4 3 2 1

10	Требования данного вида спорта понятны и близки моим внутренним убеждениям и ценностям	The requirements of this sport are clear and close to my inner beliefs and values	10 9 8 7 6 5 4 3 2 1
11	Занимаюсь уже давно, привык, ничего другого не умею	I'm engaged in this activity for a long time. I got used to, and cannot do anything else	10 9 8 7 6 5 4 3 2 1
12	Способствует организованности, в том числе и в повседневной жизни	Contributes to the organization, including everyday life	10 9 8 7 6 5 4 3 2 1
13	Высокий престиж побед в крупных соревнованиях	High prestige of victories in major competitions	10 9 8 7 6 5 4 3 2 1
14	Спорт высших достижений способ материального и финансового обеспечения себя и своей семьи	Sport of the highest achievements as a way of material and financial support for myself and my family	10 9 8 7 6 5 4 3 2 1
15	Возможность попасть в состав национальной сборной и представлять свою страну на международных соревнованиях	The opportunity to join the national team and represent my country at international competitions	10 9 8 7 6 5 4 3 2 1
16	Стремление совершенствовать свои способности, нет предела совершенства	The desire to improve my abilities, there is no limit to perfection	10 9 8 7 6 5 4 3 2 1
17	Чтобы после окончания карьеры игрока попробовать себя в качестве тренера	To try myself as a coach after retiring as a player	10 9 8 7 6 5 4 3 2 1
18	Чтобы получить специальность и стать спортивным чиновником для продвижения своего вида спорта, сделать его популярным	To get a specialty and become a sports official to promote this sport, make it popular	10 9 8 7 6 5 4 3 2 1
19	Потому что это красивый вид спорта	Because this kind of sport is very beautiful	10 9 8 7 6 5 4 3 2 1
20	Чтобы иметь больше друзей и товарищей	To have more friends	10 9 8 7 6 5 4 3 2 1
21	Расширить свой кругозор и мировоззрение	To broaden my horizons and outlook	10 9 8 7 6 5 4 3 2 1
22	Мне приятно, когда хвалит и одобряет тренер	I am pleased when the coach praises and approves me	10 9 8 7 6 5 4 3 2 1
23	Потому, что спортивный зал (спортивная база) близко (—а) от дома	Sports hall (sports facilities) is close to my house	10 9 8 7 6 5 4 3 2 1
24	Это такой вид спорта, где можно тренироваться индивидуально, независимо от других	This is a sport where you can train individually, regardless of others	10 9 8 7 6 5 4 3 2 1
25	Желание быть среди лучших и выдающихся спортсменов	Desire to be one of the best and outstanding athletes	10 9 8 7 6 5 4 3 2 1
26	Желание стать мастером спорта (мастером спорта международного класса)	Desire to become a master of sports (master of sports of international class)	10 9 8 7 6 5 4 3 2 1

27	Семейная традиция, родители (брат или сестра) занимались спортом	Family tradition, parents (brother or sister) are engaged in sports	10 9 8 7 6 5 4 3 2 1
28	Приятно испытывать чувство выполненного долга перед товарищами по команде	It's nice to feel a sense of accomplishment in front of teammates	10 9 8 7 6 5 4 3 2 1
29	Приятно, когда спортсменов показывают по телевидению, когда о них говорят по радио, пишут в газетах и журналах	It's nice when athletes are shown on television, when people talk about them on the radio, in newspapers and magazines	10 9 8 7 6 5 4 3 2 1
30	Нравится присутствие на соревнованиях родственников, друзей, товарищей, которые болеют за меня и восхищаются достигнутыми успехами	I like when my relatives, friends support me and admire my achievements	10 9 8 7 6 5 4 3 2 1
31	Чтобы бросить дурные привычки, порвать с дурной компанией, отдалиться от улицы	To quit bad habits, break with bad company, move away from the street	10 9 8 7 6 5 4 3 2 1
32	Чтобы быстрее восстановиться после перенесенной болезни (травмы)	To recover quickly from illness (injury)	10 9 8 7 6 5 4 3 2 1
33	Приятно испытывать радость побед	It's nice to experience the joy of the victory	10 9 8 7 6 5 4 3 2 1
34	Считаю, что только в этом виде спорта смогу достичь значительных успехов	I believe that only in this sport I will be able to achieve significant success	10 9 8 7 6 5 4 3 2 1
35	Пригласил заниматься тренер	My coach invited me to join the team	10 9 8 7 6 5 4 3 2 1
36	Чтобы оправдать надежды, возлагаемые на меня тренером, родителями	To live up to the hopes of my coach, parents	10 9 8 7 6 5 4 3 2 1
37	Чтобы быть более привлекательным для противоположного пола	To be more attractive to the opposite sex	10 9 8 7 6 5 4 3 2 1
38	Потому что занятия спортом повышают чувство собственного достоинства	Because doing sports increases self-esteem	10 9 8 7 6 5 4 3 2 1
39	Желание стать чемпионом страны, Европы, мира и Паралимпийских игр	Desire to become the champion of the country, Europe, the world and Paralympic games	10 9 8 7 6 5 4 3 2 1
40	Желание стать лидером, капитаном команды	Desire to become a leader, a captain of the team	10 9 8 7 6 5 4 3 2 1

Table 1.
Questionnaire of highly qualified athletes involved in five-a-side blind football.

important" (1–2 points). Three motives scored an equal low average (X) value: "To get a specialty and become a sports official to promote this sport, make it popular"; "Sports hall (sports facilities) is close to my house"; "I like when my relatives, friends support me and admire my achievements"—2.538. Also included in this

Rank of relevance	Questionnaire number	Motives of qualified athletes	Average score, X (points)	Standard error, m (points)	Median, Me (points)	Mode, Mo (points)	Standard deviation, σ (points)
1	14	Sport of the highest achievements as a way of material and financial support for myself and my family	9462	0.27	10	10	0.97
2	33	It's nice to experience the joy of the victory	9000	0.30	9	10	1.08
3	2	Your motive is achievement of success which is constantly supported by intermediate achievements: a goal, a victory, a medal	8769	0.32	9	10	1.17
4	13	High prestige of victories in major competitions	8769	0.39	9	10	1.42
5	15	The opportunity to join the national team and represent my country at international competitions	8692	0.36	9	10	1.32
6	4	Improvement of personal qualities such as endurance, will, mutual assistance, patience	8385	0.31	8	8	1.12
7	3	Develops character, mental and physical qualities	8077	0.33	8	8	1.19
8	39	Desire to become the champion of the country, Europe, the world and Paralympic games	7846	0.82	10	10	2.94
9	28	It's nice to feel a sense of accomplishment in front of teammates	7615	0.38	8	8	1.39
10	16	The desire to improve my abilities, there is no limit to perfection	7538	0.62	8	10	2.22
11	8	The opportunity to express yourself, your abilities, skills, personal qualities	7154	0.32	7	8	1.14
12	26	Desire to become a master of sports (master of sports of international class)	6692	0.80	7	10	2.87
13	25	Desire to be one of the best and outstanding athletes	6538	0.78	7	5	2.82
14	22	I am pleased when the coach praises and approves me	5846	0.72	5	5	2.61
15	12	Contributes to the organization, including everyday life	5769	0.52	6	5	1.88
16	7	A way to meet the need for new sensations, and the desire to prove that you are capable to do more	5692	0.38	6	5	1.38

Rank of relevance	Questionnaire number	Motives of qualified athletes	Average score, X (points)	Standard error, m (points)	Median, Me (points)	Mode, Mo (points)	Standard deviation, σ (points)
17	38	Because doing sports increases self-esteem	5692	0.73	6	6	2.63
18	36	To live up to the hopes of my coach, parents	5538	0.62	7	7	2.22
19	5	You like the process of sports training and its components: training, training camps, friendly games, control competitions, etc.	5308	0.29	5	5	1.03
20	1	You are always in a state of physical or emotional stress	5154	0.54	5	5	1.95
21	37	To be more attractive to the opposite sex	5154	0.64	5	6	2.30
22	11	I'm engaged in this activity for a long time. I got used to, and cannot do anything else	4923	0.55	4	4	1.98
23	34	I believe that only in this sport I will be able to achieve	4846	0.42	5	5	1.52
24	32	To recover quickly from illness (injury)	4769	0.39	5	5	1.42
25	35	My coach invited me to join the team	4615	0.83	4	3	2.99
26	40	Desire to become a leader, a captain of the team	4538	0.78	4	1	2.82
27	27	Family tradition, parents (brother or sister) are engaged in sports	4462	0.90	5	1	3.26
28	9	The ability to throw out emotions, relieve nervous and mental tension	4385	0.29	4	4	1.04
29	10	The requirements of this sport are clear and close to my inner beliefs and values	4154	0.61	5	5	2.19
30	24	This is a sport where you can train individually, regardless of others	4077	0.58	3	3	2.10
31	29	It's nice when athletes are shown on television, when people talk about them on the radio, in newspapers and magazines	4077	0.43	4	3	1.55
32	19	Because this kind of sport is very beautiful	4000	0.38	4	4	1.35
33	20	To have more friends	3846	0.77	3	2	2.79

Rank of relevance	Questionnaire number	Motives of qualified athletes	Average score, X (points)	Standard error, m (points)	Median, Me (points)	Mode, Mo (points)	Standard deviation, σ (points)
34	17	To try myself as a coach after retiring as a player	3615	0.65	4	1	2.33
35	21	To broaden my horizons and outlook	3615	0.77	2	2	2.79
36	6	Approval and support from important people for me: relatives, friends, other close people	3462	0.43	3	3	1.56
37	31	To quit bad habits, break with bad company, move away from the street	2923	0.45	3	1	1.61
38	18	To get a specialty and become a sports official to promote this sport, make it popular	2538	0.62	2	1	2.22
39	23	Sports hall (sports facilities) is close to my house	2538	0.40	3	1	1.45
40	30	I like when my relatives, friends support me and admire my achievements	2538	0.43	2	1	1.56

Table 2.
The results of mathematical and statistical processing of data on the motives of highly qualified Russian players involved in five-a-side blind football from the point of view of athletes (according to the results of the survey $n = 13$).

category is the motive "To quit bad habits, break with bad company, move away from the street" with an average of 2.923. Values of mode (Mo) in the group of motives "Absolutely not important"—1 point, medians (Me)—2–3 points; the standard error (m) from 0.40 to 0.62 indicates the unanimity of the opinion of the athletes and the regularity of falling of these motives in the category of "absolutely not important".

The motive group "Not very important" (3–4 points) is the largest, 15 motives from the average value of 3.462 ("Approval and support from important people for me: relatives, friends, other close people") to 4.923 ("I'm engaged in this activity for a long time. I got used to, and can't do anything else"). The group is characterized by equal values of analytical indicators: mode from 1 to 5 points, median—2-5 points, standard deviation (σ) does not exceed the value of 3.26 points, and the error is not more than 0.9 points. The homogeneity of the motives of this group under consideration is confirmed by the indicators of excess (Ex) and asymmetry (As) close to the symmetric distribution. The motive group "Quite important" (5–6 points) consists of 10 motives from 5.154 ("To be more attractive to the opposite sex") to 6.692 ("Desire to become a master of sports (master of sports of international class)"). The group is characterized by a symmetrical distribution, close points of the mean, mode and median. The values of the standard deviation and standard error also do not stand out from the general trend. Everything speaks of the homogeneity of the motives in question and the same opinion of the respondents regarding them.

The motives category (7–8 points) included motives with an average score of 7.154–8.769 (indicated by increasing average value): "The opportunity to express yourself, your abilities, skills, personal qualities", "The desire to improve my abilities, there is no limit to perfection", "It's nice to feel a sense of accomplishment in front of teammates", "Desire to become the champion of the country, Europe, the world and Paralympic games", "Develops character, mental and physical qualities", "Improvement of personal qualities such as endurance, will, mutual assistance, patience", "The opportunity to join the national team and represent my country at international competitions", "High prestige of victories in major competitions" and "Your motive is achievement of success which is constantly supported by intermediate achievements: a goal, a victory, a medal". Despite a slight divergence of motives in terms of analytical indicators in each individual case, the general characteristic of their homogeneity and regularity of attribution to this group remains.

The most significant and relevant motives for the respondents-players of the Russian national team (9–10 points) were the motive "It's nice to experience the joy of the victory" with average value of 9.0 and the motive "Sport of the highest achievements as a way of material and financial support for myself and my family"-9.462. In both cases, the median and mode correspond to the average score, the standard deviation is close to unity, and the error showed no more than 0.3 points. The exponents of the symmetric distribution of Ex and As are close to the normal distribution (**Table 2**).

3. Conclusions

Summarizing the results, it should be emphasized the homogeneity and the same attitude of the Russian national team players to the motives proposed in the questionnaire to engage in five-a-side blind football. The values of the totality of analytical indicators reinforce the conclusion about the regularity of ranking and classifying each motive in the corresponding category of significance.

In this regard, the relevance of developing and improving the methodology for sports training of qualified 5 × 5 (B1) football players (sports of the blind) is beyond doubt.

Summing up the research attention should be paid to homogeneity and collective opinion regarding the group of motives of each significance category. Analytical calculations confirm this thesis. The survey results suggest that highly qualified.

Paralympic blind football players, possessing significant baggage of competitive experience, mainly international, are aware of the significant requirements of the sport in question, appreciating the importance of the correct way to prepare an athlete.

In accordance with this, the sports training of highly qualified Paralympic blind football players should be determined by the scientific and methodological content and be based on the international best practices of the best teams in organizing the sports training process.

Such an approach will allow not only high-class athletes to realize their potential and achieve the highest results, but also less qualified players to improve their skills and become candidates for joining the national team of the country in the future.

Acknowledgements

I would like to thank everyone who participated and continues to participate in the study of the problems of Paralympic futsal (blind sports) in Russia. First of all, I would like to mention the doctor of pedagogical sciences, professor and part-time colleague of mine in five-a-side blind football sports team of the Russian Federation Alexander Makhov for valuable advice, guidance, experience in preparing and organizing scientific activities. My friend, chief and also colleague on the Russian national team, Pechenin Kirill, who supports me in my initiatives, provides a basis for research on the above topics.

I also express my respect for the work to the head coach of the Russian national team Alexander Nikolaevich Erastov, in which the team became the European champion in 2017, as well as to the head of the team Sputnov Valery Vasilyevich for unlimited optimism and imagination.

Author details

Konstantin Popenko
Yoshkar-Ola, Republic of Mari El, Russia

*Address all correspondence to: minsport.popenko@yandex.ru

References

[1] The Second Section of the All-Russian Register of Sports [Internet]. 2019. Available from: https://www.minsport.gov.ru/2018/VRVS_07092018.xls [Accessed: 07 August 2019]

[2] Makhov AS. Adaptive Sport in Russia and Abroad: Formation, Organization, Regulation: Monograph. Moscow: RUDN University; 2011. 196p

[3] Abramova LP editor. The program for the development of sports for the blind in the Russian Federation for 2013-2020. Moscow: LLC Sports and Athletic Organization Federation of the Blind Sports; 2013. 363p

[4] The Sport of the Blind. Pioneers of disabled sports. Paralympic Sport. 2017; **3**(4). 90:35–40. Available from: http://паралимпийскийспорт.рф/upload/uf/c1a/c1ada041733523e553b86be87269c3b8.pdf

[5] Popenko KS, Makhov AS. Moderm status of mini football 5x5 (B1) (sports of blind people) in Russia. Prensa Medica Argentina. 2019;**105**(1):1-4. DOI: 10.41720032-745X.1000328

[6] Popenko KS. Problems of the development of Paralympic futsal (blind sports) in Russia by the example of the republic of Mari El. In: Materials of the VI Interregional Scientific-Practical Conference, 27 April 2018. Yoshkar-Ola: GBPOU of the Republic of Mari El "School of the Olympic reserve"; 2018. pp. 212-217

[7] Drozhalkin VA. Sports motivation as a leading factor in performance in sports and competitive activities. Modern Research and Innovation. 2015;**4**: 161-163. Available from: http://web.snauka.ru/issues/2015/04/52492 [Accessed: 18 September 2019]

[8] Popenko KS. Training motivations tests in Italian national futsal 5×5 B1 (blind sport) team. Teoriya i Praktika Fizicheskoy Kultury. 2019;**5**:22-24

[9] Kornev AV. Motivation of sports activities of students of special (correctional) schools. Theory and Practice of Physical Culture. 2016;**3**: 35-37

[10] Korneva MA. Features of motivation of athletes with disabilities with damage to the musculoskeletal system to participate in the training process in the Russian bench press. Theory and Practice of Physical Culture. 2014;**6**:37-58

[11] Kuzmin EB. Sports motivation as a mental state of an athlete's personality. Human Health, Theory and Methodology of Physical Culture and Sports. 2016;**1**:97-110

[12] Makhov AS. Evaluation of the effectiveness of the formation of motivation for physical exercises and sports in people with disabilities. Herald of a Sports Science. 2012;**3**:52-56

[13] Makhov AS. Psychological and pedagogical features of motivation for playing sports in people with visual impairment. Vestnik CHGPU Named for I. Yakovlev. 2013;**77**(1–2):120-124

[14] Rysakova OG. The meaning and structure of motives of deaf athletes of Russia and abroad to snowboarding. Scientific Notes of the P.F. Lesgaft. 2015;**124**(6):167-173

[15] Shaboltas AV. Motives for sports in the highest achievements in adolescence [Dissertation abstract]. St. Petersburg; 1998. 21p